HCG for Foodies

*Clever Cooking and Smart Science
for the HCG Diet*

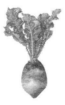

Dana Falk, Ph.D. & Kelsey Klausmeyer, N.D.

ISBN-13: 978-1-7332765-5-9

e-book ISBN: 978-1-7332765-1-1

First Edition

Library of Congress Registration TXu 2-220-051

Printed in the United States of America

Book design by Dana Falk

icmedicine.com

www.seattlesoundview.org

For my mother, Paula and my best friend, Lisa.
I wish everyone had people of such character in their life.

— DF

Dedicated to my mother, Marilyn and my sister, Bre.

— KK

SPECIAL THANKS

Brandon Chan
Katy Gronowski
Naomi Guilbert
Hiroshi Koshiyama
MaryBeth Sabine
Bob Stremba

HCG for Foodies

*Clever Cooking
and
Smart Science*

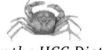

for the HCG Diet

Contents

Disclaimer

This book is intended as a reference volume only. The information presented herein is not intended to diagnose, treat, cure or prevent any disease. This book is not intended as a substitute for any treatment prescribed by your healthcare professional. The authors offer no medical or psychological assessment nor any clinical intervention.

Full clearance from your healthcare team is recommended prior to initiating or modifying any diet or lifestyle program. Your licensed medical provider should be apprised of any nutritional changes you have made and consulted regarding any changes you wish to make. If you suspect you have a medical condition, please seek competent medical care.

The authors do not guarantee, warrantee, represent or promise that any information presented herein will result in the maintenance, improvement or resolution of any and all medical or psychological conditions.

The authors claim no responsibility to any person or entity for any liability, loss or damage, caused or alleged to be caused, directly or indirectly, as a result of the application or interpretation of the information herein. The authors shall not be in any way liable or responsible for any outcomes achieved or obtained by any reader of this book.

Note to Healthcare Professionals

What we refer to as "The HCG Diet" is technically a low calorie, ketogenic diet. In his 1954 treatment protocol, Dr. Albert Simeons used human chorionic gonadotropin to induce this same action — driving metabolic pathways to help the body use fat stores for fuel — though this was well before the term "nutritional ketosis" was in common use.

HCG is not a fad diet, when medically supervised. Rather, it's pharmacotherapy with a naturally occurring human hormone that induces ketosis. This, in combination with behavioral medicine, comprises the HCG Diet. Some patients with existing hormonal imbalance may not respond well to the medication. Patients should be monitored closely — every 1-2 weeks is advised — while on the hormone treatment. Menstrual irregularity, allergic reactions and infection at the injection site have been observed.

The original protocol did not include MCT oil. We are proponents of dispensing high-quality MCT oil to patients for prevention of constipation, gall stones and kidney stones. The use of electrolytes and multivitamins is also encouraged, to offset any deficiencies the low-calorie phase may induce.

The ketogenic diet (also referred to as Low Carb/High Fat or LCHF) is an evidence-based, empirically supported treatment, proven effective for remitting Type II diabetes, provided it has not yet progressed to kidney disease (Fung, 2016). Your patients who continue with a ketogenic diet beyond the HCG treatment protocol are likely to maintain their weight loss. That is, when back to normal caloric intake, if they practice a diet low in carbohydrate (less than 20-30g per day) moderate in protein (.8 - 1.5 grams of protein per pound of lean body mass) and if they eat healthy fats to satiety (avoiding vegetable oils and other PUFAs) they should maintain weight lost while on HCG (McKenzie, Hallberg & Creighton, 2017).

Newly diagnosed diabetics benefit from a diet low in carbohydrate. Patel, et. al. (2016) found that reductions in glucose, driven by reductions in weight, delayed progressive metabolic worsening with this population. Dietary changes effectively mitigated hyperglycemia in this peer-reviewed study.

Patients who return to the standard American diet, which is relatively high in carbohydrate, tend to return to a state of hyperinsulinemia and thus more easily regain the weight they have lost.

It takes time in every discipline for clinical practice to reflect current research; this is particularly true when a paradigm shift is required. Some healthcare providers and some weight loss programs continue to recommend a low-fat diet for weight loss, though randomized clinical trials have established that carbohydrate intake, not fat consumption, drives hyperinsulinemia, NAFLD and adiposopathy. Thus, we now know that dietary fat is not what drives obesity (Volek & Phinney, 2012.)

Where practice *does* reflect current research on nutritional ketosis, patient outcomes are remarkable. At the Duke University *Lifestyle Medicine Clinic,* for example, patient reversals of biomarkers for Type II Diabetes have garnered so much attention that other teaching hospitals are modeling their obesity treatment protocols after the clinic at Duke.

Current research corroborates the outcomes observed at Duke: nutritional ketosis has proven effective for treatment of metabolic syndrome. Hallberg, et. al. (2018) found that at the one year mark, subjects consuming a low carb/high fat (LCHF) diet lost significantly more weight than subjects on a low fat/high carb diet did — even when calories consumed was controlled for. Most significant is the finding that patients on a ketogenic diet also decreased significantly on inflammatory markers such as C-Reactive Protein and white blood cell count (p = <.001.)

The ketogenic diet also confers the advantage of much higher long-term patient compliance than standard low fat/high carbohydrate diets do (83% compliance at the one year mark; N = 286). This finding contradicts the assumption that most patients cannot maintain a low carbohydrate lifestyle. Measuring the subject's β-hydroxybutyrate levels across the first year confirmed that they were producing ketone bodies. That is, subjects didn't just *self-report* compliance with a low carbohydrate regimen, they produced clinical evidence that subjects *had complied* with a low carb diet (Hallberg, et. al., 2018.)

We believe that the HCG protocol may facilitate significant weight loss and that following this up with a ketogenic diet is indicated for patients who wish to continue gradual weight loss. Highly recommended reading for both patients and providers is "Keto." (2018) by Maria Emmerich and Craig Emmerich. This book is an exceptional resource for orienting both patients and providers to the science and practice of nutritional ketosis.

HCG for Foodies in a Nutshell

This book is for people who want to maximize their weight loss while on the HCG Diet but who are concerned that their passion for food, culture and cooking could undermine their ability to stick with it. This diet is quite challenging and tremendously rewarding. We think that strategizing will be worth your while.

Our recommendations are focused on your health first, then logical food choices, then creative cooking. We believe that we improve upon the original HCG protocol using the current science of fat metabolism. Happily, approaching the HCG Diet scientifically will give you far more food choices that facilitate weight loss.

We also believe that having precise recipes is not the key to success here. We think that clever hacks for flavorful cooking when faced with limited ingredients is more the point. *HCG for Foodies* is not a classic cookbook; it's a guide to kicking ass on the HCG Diet using endocrinology, psychology and finesse in the kitchen.

We offer ideas for your creative cooking in a variety of ways. There are (1) *traditional recipes* with detailed instructions; (2) *casual recipe ideas and flavor combinations*, as well as (3) *suggested ingredients and products*. The casual recipe ideas, flavor combinations and suggested ingredients appear in bold, since they are all tucked within the text. The traditional recipes are each featured on individual pages, so they're not hard to find.

We call your attention to products our patients find helpful, but new products hit the market all the time. In the two years it took to write this book, for example, a great many new beverages made without sugar or artificial sweeteners became available. We encourage you to apply what you learn about HCG-safe ingredients and do some looking of your own.

New criticisms of existing products come to light, too. If you learn something compelling that is evidence-based about any of the ingredients we describe here, go with the most recent intelligence. This is a process!

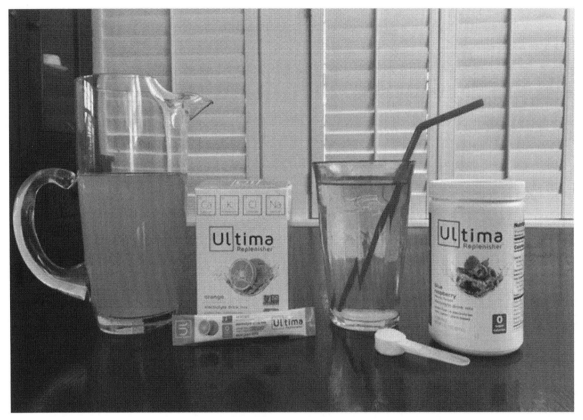

Photo: Dana Falk

Ultima Replenisher electrolyte drink mix came to our attention just as we went to press. These drinks are made with HCG-safe sweeteners, have no calories and taste great! We recommend this product, but can't predict what time will tell about it or any of products we discuss, with regard to their usefulness for the HCG Diet.

You'll notice that the dishes photographed do not look professional; that's because they're not. *HCG for Foodies* began as a strategies manual for our patients. We want to share as many tools for success as possible, even if they are home grown and down-to-earth rather than professional, studio quality.

Professional Healthcare during HCG

Doing HCG with the help of a book is very good; doing it with the expertise of a medical provider is even better. Naturopathic Doctors (NDs) are in an excellent position to guide you with a ketogenic diet like HCG. If your insurance list does not include NDs, they may still be covered by your insurance, out of network. Go to naturopathic.org if you need help locating a Naturopathic Physician in your area.

Any healthcare provider who has been trained in Functional Medicine would be great to work with while on HCG. Nurse Practitioners (ARNP), Medical Doctors (MD), Doctors of Osteopathic Medicine (DO), Physician Assistants (PA), Naturopathic Doctors (ND) and Pharmacists (MPharm, PharmD) are among the professionals who may complete specialized, accredited training in Functional Medicine.

These are all providers who have a strong interest in how and why illness occurs — in root causes, not just symptoms. Functional Medicine practitioners embrace the complexity of genetic, biochemical and lifestyle explanations for illness and they personalize their treatment plan to each patient. They will likely understand nutritional ketosis, which would put you in capable hands. For help finding a healthcare provider who is certified in Functional Medicine, go to www.IFM.org.

Quick Start to the Ketogenic Diet

The goal of the HCG Diet is to utilize deep ketosis to access stored fat. This is also the goal of the ketogenic diet. People who "eat keto" shift their body from burning sugar for energy to burning fat by sharply reducing carbohydrate intake.

While on the HCG Diet, patients take the human chorionic gonadotropin (HCG) hormone to facilitate a deep state of ketosis extremely efficiently. Although the HCG Diet is a brief treatment and the ketogenic diet a lifestyle, completing a round of HCG creates a more powerful start to nutritional ketosis than gradual dietary changes can accomplish.

The HCG Diet targets fat loss. The ketogenic diet on the other hand offers vast health benefits beyond weight loss — people "eat keto" to treat diabetes or epilepsy, to reduce inflammation and joint pain, to sharpen their mental clarity, reduce their appetite, cravings and acid reflux or to improve their sleep and complexion. With or without an interest in weight loss, people must be in a deep state of ketosis to reap these other health benefits.

We also observe clinically that HCG may reduce carbohydrate cravings. We don't yet have the randomized clinical trials to solidify these observations, but it's worth noting that this is a benefit some patients report with HCG. Reduced carb intake is both the mechanism that drives ketosis and one benefit of it. It makes sense that HCG would operate in this same way.

In all, using the HCG Diet as a springboard to the ketogenic diet makes perfect sense. If it's something you will do, take your time with HCG Phase 3, when you are gradually adding fats back to your diet. Being in ketosis is more about eating low carbohydrate than it is about eating high fat, but it's common for people on keto to eat a good amount of healthy fat. Be certain your gall bladder is ready for this by rebuilding your tolerance for fatty acids gradually during Phase 3.

There's more detail about the transition from HCG to Keto in a separate section, called "Continuing a Ketogenic Lifestyle." You'll find this information at the tail end of our discussion of HCG Phase 3.

What is a Foodie?

We're thinking of foodies as people for whom food is sensual and multi-dimensional. The primary issue is not just over-eating. Foodies adore learning about cultures through cuisine. They try new restaurants even if it's inconvenient, enjoy shopping in specialty markets, seek out the best meat, fish and cheese. Foodies improvise their own dishes and improve upon recipes. They enjoy reading cookbooks, learning technique and trying kitchen tools that present new possibilities. Foodies are people who consider culinary choices an important part of their identity; they love many things about food, not just eating it.

Meals should be delicious and special for foodies, not just familiar or filling. Since their palate is quite discerning, some overeat and some do not. We aren't in love with the word "foodie," but we think it captures nicely that multi-dimensional relationship with exploration, culture, cooking and eating that we're after.

Our goal with *HCG for Foodies* is to enable readers to use their affinity for flavor, food and culture to their *benefit* during HCG Phase 2, when their choices and calories are limited — rather than allowing their good taste to undermine them.

Not Just for Foodies

If you couldn't care less about cooking and just want to know how to maximize your weight loss while on HCG, this book is for you, too. We offer cooking and mental health insights along the way, but we also just teach you what to do. You'll learn methods for choosing your own fruits, vegetables and proteins, for example, but you will also see lists of recommended foods that have already been calculated for you.

HCG for Foodies is not a "cookbook" in the traditional sense. It's a guide for the HCG Diet that's about strategy — and recipes are one of those strategies. We arm you with ingredients, flavor combinations, dishes, snacks and cooking techniques that will render satisfying meals. In a few cases we provide detailed recipes, but more often we provide the ingredients and method but not precise measurements.

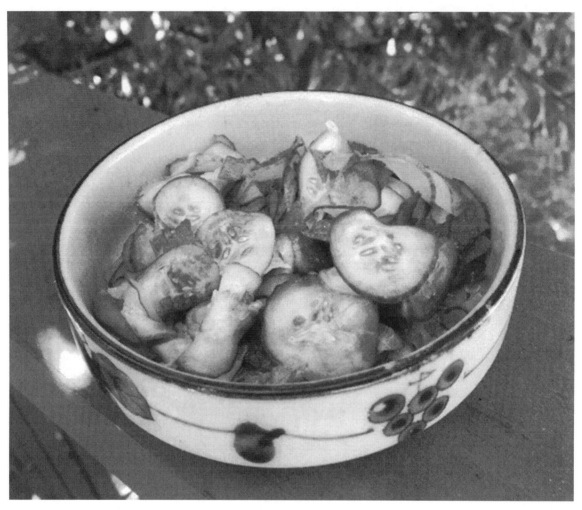

Photo: Dana Falk

Some of our recipes are very precise, but most look like this direction for Japanese cucumber salad (sunomono): Thinly sliced cucumber + rice vinegar + sweetener to taste + pinch salt + (optional) chopped fresh mint or grated fresh ginger. Leave cucumbers in vinegar marinade for at least an hour. Drain well, but save marinade. Serve chilled. Try cold, sliced prawns on top. We offer the idea, you run with it.

This is the way most foodies like to cook — with inspiration rather than precision — but if you personally prefer structure, this may drive you a little crazy. We're confident you'll find other kinds of vital information here, designed to minimize your suffering and maximize your results while on HCG.

We offer three kinds of practical information:

1. Scientific Insights

A little endocrinology never hurt anyone, especially those who want their decisions to be guided by a solid understanding of how their body responds to what they eat while on HCG.

2. Cooking Ideas

Suggested ingredients, flavor combinations, dishes and cooking strategies that stimulate your creativity and improve your stamina for the low-calorie phase.

3. Psychological Insights

Research and experience with patients means we know how people create lasting change and what challenges them. We break it down and offer opportunities for self-assessment.

HCG for Foodies was originally created for our patients in Seattle. It's written by Dr. Kelsey Klausmeyer, a Naturopathic Physician who specializes in the treatment of obesity and Dr. Dana Falk, a Licensed Psychologist who specializes in adult transitions and mechanisms of change. Joining forces across disciplines has cultivated a richer menu of strategies for your success than we could have created as individuals.

We hope that our pleasure working successfully with patients on the HCG Diet offers you the nitty-gritty details you'll need to accomplish your goals. We know this process is partly about trust.

Our Recommendations

We are heavily focused on strategies for a pleasant and successful Phase 2 (P2.) This is the part of the HCG Diet in which you'll be targeting the number of calories your provider recommends (generally, 500-800 calories per day) and eating a limited range of foods. You will be eating as low in fat and carbs as possible, so you'll need to be quite creative about getting flavor and texture in your meals. When you have so few degrees of freedom, we believe every morsel of information and inspiration can be a tremendous help.

For example, one patient told us that learning about the availability of grated lemongrass in the frozen food case made a big difference for him. This person loves Southeast Asian flavors. He was able to add Pho Noodle soup, lemongrass grilled prawns and chicken larb in lettuce cups to his repertoire, which made the diet far easier for him. Another patient told us that she had not realized how ambivalent she was about eating differently. Working through the *Twenty Preparations for HCG* and *How Behavior Change Works* sections of the book enabled her to examine how she'd actually been avoiding losing weight. On her next round of HCG, she was finally able step on the gas, because she was no longer ambivalent about succeeding.

Hormones exert powerful influences in the body and negative side effects are possible. Some women experience hormonal shifts and menstrual cycle irregularity, for example. Side effects vary widely in response to dosage and timing. It's ideal to use HCG with the guidance of a healthcare provider if you can.

Prescribing human chorionic gonadotropin for appetite and weight loss is off-label, meaning that it is not yet FDA-approved for this purpose (though there is growing evidence for this use of it). On-label, HCG is typically used in fertility treatments for both men and women. In men, it may also be prescribed to treat low testosterone. When prescribed for fertility, doses are far greater than when prescribed for obesity. A typical fertility dose for women would be 10,000 IU per day. By contrast, 125-200 IU per day would most often be prescribed for patients on the HCG Diet.

Compounding pharmacies have worked successfully with the hormone — they created an effective HCG nasal spray, for example — but at the time of this writing, the Food and Drug Administration has restricted compounding of HCG. This puts manufacturing of prescription HCG in the hands of pharmaceutical companies, and the price of prescription strength HCG has increased.

Some people use over-the-counter or homeopathic formulations of HCG, which may be administered orally (sublingual tablets or liquid drops), nasally or by injection. Of these, we recommend the injections, if used with caution. Look into the source if purchasing non-prescription forms of HCG. It's possible these formulations may be a few molecules of the hormone in a solution, rather than pure hormone. The theory is that the hormone's energetic information is transferred to the body and will have an effect similar to the pure hormone.

Once on the diet, **your biggest challenge may be dealing with other people.** Don't skip the sections "Factor in Social Expectations" and "Interpersonal Skills for Transitions" in this book. Few people are fully prepared to deal with the attention, questions, concerns, challenges and hurt feelings that may occur when they are in the process of change. Even when people are quite enthusiastic about with you're doing, it may feel a bit weird to talk about. Especially tend to these sections of the book if you're the type who hates to inconvenience others or are reluctant to call attention to yourself.

For some people, the biggest challenge is not other people expecting them to eat, it's their own ambivalence about dieting or becoming slender. These thoughts are almost always either unconscious, or just partially conscious. There are perfectly good reasons people *think they are certain* they want to be smaller, and want work towards that, but deep down have reservations. Read the section "Why People Fear Weight Loss" for a very long list of these reasons; it may help you to pinpoint any unconscious sticking points and thus prevent rebellion.

We also offer guidelines for the Loading Phase (which precedes the low calorie phase) and for HCG Phase 3 (which follows it). We want you to lose the most weight possible and to keep it off to the best of your ability.

Central to *HCG for Foodies* is the perspective that there are foods on the original HCG protocol you probably shouldn't eat and a huge variety foods you *can* eat that aren't on that protocol. The issue while on HCG is the carbohydrate and fat content of your choices. **We recommend no more than 20 grams total carbohydrate per day, with the goal being as few carbs as possible while still eating some veggies.**

Dr. Albert Simeons wrote *Pounds and Inches* in 1954 to describe a treatment he used with hospital patients in Rome. We know more than we did back then about the mechanisms of weight loss on HCG, but you should make an independent decision about whether you'd like to adhere to the original Simeons protocol or to incorporate the advances we note here. We describe both approaches to the diet, in full detail, so you can follow whichever you please.

For some people, following a protocol to the letter is ideal. Structure and repetition don't bother them nearly as much as making multiple decisions would bug them. For most foodies, though, compliance would be difficult without some opportunity to improvise. Do whatever suits you.

The cooking ideas in *HCG for Foodies* are all safe for Phase 2; in fact, our suggestions are pretty conservative. If you wish for a larger number of recipes, written in traditional form with precise instructions, there exist HCG books that are entirely cookbooks.

Overview of the HCG Diet

HCG Diet Phase	Action	Purpose	Duration
Phase 1 LOADING	Eat high in fat and calories, low in carbohydrate.	Induce ketosis, in which body is fueled by its own fat rather than by glucose.	Two full days, while on the HCG hormone.
Phase 2 (P2) VERY LOW CALORIE	Eat as low in fat and carbohydrate as possible while on low calorie diet; usually 500-800 calories per day.	Pull from your stored body fat by combining low calorie/carb/fat consumption with deep ketosis.	23-40 days while on the hormone, plus 1-3 days low calorie days without HCG.
Phase 3 (P3) STABILIZING	Slowly re-introduce fats and calories. Optional: Test individual foods for food sensitivities.	Prevent weight rebound, losing ketosis and gallbladder problems.	Three weeks, or more if desired. No longer on hormone.
Phase 4	Some people refer to life after HCG as Phase 4, when you work to maintain the weight loss forever.	Not an official phase of the diet, but we end the book with a section on food as a lifelong issue and overcoming compulsive eating.	

Old Protocol and New Advances

In 1954, a British endocrinologist named Albert Simeons wrote the manuscript "Pounds and Inches." In this manuscript he described his clinical observations treating obesity patients at Salvator Mundi International Hospital in Rome. He found that when administered the human chorionic gonadotropin (HCG) hormone, patients could utilize their existing body fat at an accelerated rate. When he prescribed limited food choices and portions along with the hormone, these patients were able to lose weight very effectively.

Now, more than 65 years on, we know that he was right about the way HCG mobilizes stored fat when the patient is on a very low calorie, low fat diet. However, we believe that he was not entirely correct about some of the foods on that protocol and about mandating a rigid portion size, regardless of the food being eaten.

Understanding the Original HCG Protocol (1954)

If you're curious about the original manuscript, *Pounds and Inches* by A. T. W. Simeons is available on amazon.com in paperback and as an e-book. He offers some interesting theories about obesity, explains how HCG works to access what he calls "abnormal fat reserves" and describes how his patients responded to treatment. Dr. Simeons contributed far more than just telling patients what to eat, so our summary of his 1954 HCG protocol (below) is a bastardization of sorts; we are referring only to the "how-to" content of his manuscript. Some of his language may strike us as offensive by modern-day standards (in reference to gender roles and overweight people) but Dr. Simeons' full manuscript is a valuable read.

Here, we will cut to the chase, though. We'll show you what the Simeons protocol was, then examine it in light of the advances in nutrition science and endocrinology we now enjoy. This way, we can honor what he created while pointing out those foods on the original protocol that are not wise choices, in our opinion. Next we'll offer guidelines for selecting your own proteins, fruits and vegetables while on HCG. We think there's far more variety available to you than what appears in the original protocol.

Dr. Simeons might not have cared for our philosophy. He wrote:*"...The most tiresome patients are those who...come up with all manner of ingenious variations which they compile from their little books. When one has spent years of weary research trying to make a diet as attractive as possible...culinary geniuses who are out to improve their unhappy lot are hard to take...."*

At that time, Dr. Simeons wanted patients to adhere strictly to the protocol he designed, but we think that as a clinical scientist, he'd probably agree that new evidence should always drive treatment decisions.

Many people do follow the original HCG protocol to the letter. We recommend more contemporary, evidence-based choices, but make no mistake, you can certainly lose weight using the 1954 protocol exactly as written and many people do. It's truly up to you.

Below is a detailed summary of the diet protocol portion of *Pounds and Inches*. This is what Dr. Simeons prescribed to his patients.

Original HCG Diet Protocol (1954)

— There are 26-43 days on the diet protocol. That's 23-40 doses of HCG + three days at the end, still on a low calorie diet (800-1,000 calories) but *without* taking HCG.

— At the start of the diet, he prescribes two days of gorging on high calorie foods while taking the HCG hormone. This includes sweets, fats and refined flours. Patients are instructed to eat to the point of feeling very full, in the original protocol.

— Next, the very low calorie phase, which lasts 23 - 37 days. Patients continue taking HCG daily, but now are consuming only 500 calories per day, maximum. (Caloric intake is set at 500 on the original protocol, regardless of patient metabolic condition, goals, hunger or physical activity.)

— Patients should be reminded, Simeons writes, that taking the HCG hormone means patients are surviving more on their *stored* fat than on the 500 calories they consume.

— During the very low calorie phase, patients eat two meals per day, with only coffee or tea for breakfast. Details below.

— At each of these two meals, patients consume a maximum of 100 grams of lean protein. All visible fat is trimmed and the item is weighed prior to cooking.

— Eating 200 grams of lean protein per day is thought to facilitate maximum weight loss, as is eating a small amount of starch. The way those 500 calories are apportioned, Simeons said, is of utmost importance.

— Portion size for protein is set at 100 grams per meal, regardless of the food(s) chosen.

— Patients should drink at least two liters of water per day.

— Patients should not use any oil-based products on their skin, such as moisturizers, liquid foundation, sunscreen, coconut oil or shea butter soaps, hair products, hand or eye creams.

— No medications may be used without special permission of the physician, on the original protocol.

— Patients are instructed to choose only from the foods listed (below), regardless of their carbohydrate content.

— Patients are advised to carefully check their food choices against the diet protocol list, rather than relying upon memory.

— Patients are implored not to substitute other fruits or vegetables for those listed, even if these contain fewer calories. Simeons stated that the chemical composition of some fruits and veggies will stall weight loss.

— Patients may omit any food they wish.

— No food or calories unused on one day may be saved for the following day of the diet.

Here's what was on Simeons' original list of acceptable foods for HCG Phase 2:

The items we comment upon later, under "Advances Since the Original Protocol," are in bold.

PROTEIN
Allowed: Veal, **beef**, kidney, chicken breast, fresh white fish, lobster, crab, shrimp, crawfish.

Meat must be trimmed of all visible fat and prepared without use of fats.

Not allowed: Salmon, eel, **tuna**, herring, **all dried, smoked or pickled fish**, **eggs.**

Occasional: A patient may eat one whole egg (including yolk) if it is served with the whites of three additional eggs.

Occasionally, 100 grams of skim-milk cottage cheese may be a substitute for meat, but no other cheese is allowed.

VEGETABLES
Spinach, chard, chicory, beet greens, 'green salad,' **tomato**, celery, **fennel**, **onion**, red radishes, cucumber, asparagus, cabbage.

Vegetables that stall weight loss, according to 1954 protocol:
Okra, artichoke, pimiento (sweet red) peppers.

CRISP BREADS
One thin **breadstick** (Italian grissini) or piece of **Melba toast** per meal.

FRUIT
Full **apple**, 1/2 **orange**, 1/2 grapefruit or a "handful" of strawberries.

Eating two small apples that weigh the same as one large apple is not allowed. Only one apple is allowed per day.

The juice of one lemon is allowed per day.

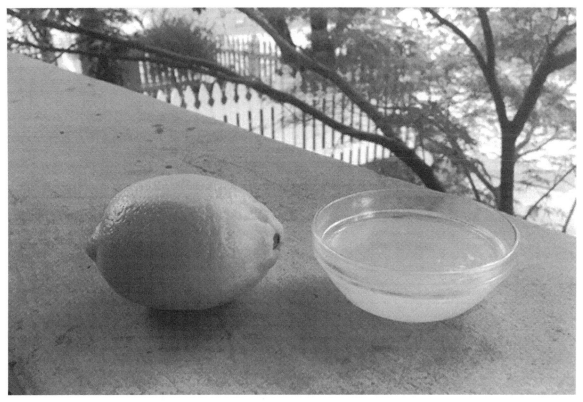

Photo: Dana Falk

The juice of a 5 oz medium lemon [left] yielded 3 tbs + 1/3 tsp of juice [right]. A really big lemon would yield about 4 tbs juice = 1/4 cup = 59 mL. So let's say Dr. Simeons approved of 3-4 tbs of lemon juice per day on HCG. Remember to roll the lemon on the countertop and microwave it 15-20 seconds to yield the most juice.

UNLIMITED CONSUMPTION
Tea and coffee, without sugar, are unlimited. Sweeteners like **saccharin** may be used. Maximum of one tablespoon of milk per day is allowed.

Plain (still) water and sparkling mineral water (seltzer) are unlimited.
All of these beverages are all allowed in unlimited quantity and at any time.

USE AS-NEEDED, FOR SEASONING
Allowed: Salt, pepper, vinegar, mustard powder, **garlic**, sweet basil, parsley, thyme, marjoram and other fresh herbs may be used for seasoning.

Not allowed: Oil, butter or **"dressing."**

Any food not listed above is forbidden on the original 1954 protocol. Dr. Simeons stated *"...the patient is assured that nothing permissible [to eat] has been left out...."*

How to compose your meals, according to the 1954 HCG protocol:

BREAKFAST
No food is consumed.
Unlimited tea and coffee may be consumed. No sugar allowed, but sweeteners such as **saccharin** may be used. Maximum one tablespoon of milk per day.

LUNCH
100 grams of protein from the list above, weighed before cooking.
One serving of vegetables.
One serving of fruit.
One crisp bread of choice (breadstick or Melba toast).

No more than four items from the list of acceptable foods may be eaten at any one meal.

DINNER

Precisely the same instructions as for lunch.

BETWEEN MEALS

Patients may eat as many times **throughout the day** as they wish. There is no requirement that food be consumed in just two sittings, like a traditional lunch and dinner.

Dr. Simeons noted *"...There is no objection to breaking up the two meals, for instance having a breadstick and an apple for breakfast or before going to bed, provided they are deducted from the regular meals...."*

However, patients may have only one serving of crisp bread or fruit at a time. The second serving must be consumed at another time of day.

So that's the scoop on the original, Simeons HCG diet protocol from 1954. Next, we present our recommendations, which respect this protocol but add modern ketogenic science.

Advances Since the Original Protocol

Below are updates to the original protocol that we believe current science and practice support. We recommend you observe these guidelines as amendments to the 1954 protocol.

<u>Under general instructions for the diet protocol</u>

We do not agree that precisely 500 calories is the recommended caloric intake for all patients, though it is right for some people.

It's absolutely true that patients must consume very low calories while on HCG — otherwise the body would not need to pull from its stored fat, of course — but most healthcare providers managing HCG patients consider basal metabolic rate, patient's ability to remain on the diet, amount of weight that person has to lose and several other factors when determining a patient's caloric goals. Generally, 500-800 calories is what's prescribed, not 500 calories on the nose, for all patients.

We recommend that you count not just calories but grams of carbohydrate. Veggies have carbs (in fact they *are* carbs) so we do not recommend that you avoid carbohydrates entirely. **We recommend you do eat vegetables, but keep your carbohydrate intake as low as possible, with a maximum of 20 grams total carbs per day.** This is to protect your being in ketosis.

Under breakfast in the original protocol

You may eat breakfast if you would like to. There's no requirement that you have only tea or coffee in the morning. It's to your benefit to delay your first food of the day, if you can, because you're delaying your first insulin response of the day, but there's no rule about skipping breakfast.

Saccharin is mentioned under breakfast. That's just one artificial sweetener, but *all* artificial sweeteners should be avoided, in our opinion. In modern terms, that would mean avoiding products like Sweet n' Low, Splenda and Equal. If you need sweetness in your coffee, use an "alternative natural sweetener" like stevia, stevia glycerite, monk fruit extract, allulose, erythritol, xylitol or some combination of these (which is quite common). There's much more about each of these options in the "Alternative Natural Sweeteners" section of the book.

Under fruits listed in the original protocol

Apples and oranges we do not recommend. There are some fantastic uses for the zest, pith and membrane of citrus fruits, but eating half an orange or a whole apple would not be wise while on HCG, in our opinion. These high-glycemic fruits have more carbohydrate than Melba toast and bread sticks do!

If you will be following the original protocol to the letter (thus eating apples and oranges on P2) try hard to use them as *flavoring* in your cooking rather than eating them as whole fruit. There are fruits that have far less sugar than apples and orange do; why not focus on them? You'll see how to identify these safer fruits and a list of our suggestions under "Method for Choosing Fruit and Vegetables."

Strawberries and grapefruit are mentioned in the original protocol and are fine in small amounts. Some people limit their fruit to "berries only" while on HCG. Although on average, berries are lower in sugar and higher in fiber than most fruits are, not all of them are low carbohydrate choices. For example, blueberries are not one of the fruits lowest in carbohydrate, but raspberries are. We really encourage you to make your choices intentional, based upon the 20 grams carbohydrate maximum per day, rather than by ruling an entire category in or out.

Under crisp breads listed in the original protocol

The Melba toast and grissini bread sticks on the original protocol are not recommended. Some patients say that eating bread sticks or Melba toast on P2 increases their cravings or their overall hunger, but the primary reason we don't recommend them is that they are high in carbohydrate without other phytonutrients to bring some benefit.

The starch in bread sticks and such instruct your body to release insulin. Insulin is a hormonal message to the body to *store* fat, not burn it. In short, starches counteract ketosis. Getting your body "into ketosis" is precisely what the HCG hormone accomplishes that is so special.

Can you make one breadstick per day work for HCG if it's important to you? Yes, it would probably mean no fruit and only the lowest-carb veggies for the day, but if you can bring total carbs in under 20 grams, yes, you can do it.

There is now low carb Melba toast on the market, for example *Carbolicious* brand. Regular Melba toast has about 13 total carbs per 17 g serving. Carbolicious has 3 total carbs for a 15 g serving. Remember though: 20 g total carbohydrate per day is not our suggested amount, it's our suggested *maximum*. Eating fewer carbs, while including vegetables, is best for weight loss.

Thus, if you want to crush a breadstick to use as a crunchy coating for fish, why not choose a lower carb cracker for that purpose, like Finn Crisp, which has 5g carb per cracker, or Wasa Thins, which have 5.5 g carbs per cracker? *There's no magic to Melba toast or grissini*; you can improve upon those choices if you wish to.

Under seasonings in the original protocol

Dr. Simeons cautions against the use of "dressings," but his protocol was written before the use of MCT oil. We do allow — in fact recommend — that patients use MCT oil to concoct salad dressings, dipping sauces, moisture for tuna, chicken salad and such. Our patients say that being able to create a dressing with MCT oil that tastes really good is crucial to their being able to stick with the diet. Check out the section "Tricks with Alternative Natural Sweeteners" for some dressing ideas.

Under "between meals" in the original protocol

Research shows that people lose weight more effectively if they eat fewer times each day. The body releases insulin each time it must respond to food intake and insulin is the fat *storage* hormone. We believe that advising patients to consume their calories as they wish throughout the day, as Dr. Simeons did, is not the ideal strategy.

Current research also shows that people lose weight more effectively when they contain their eating to a shorter range of hours. This shorter "eating window" produces a mini fasting period between dinner time and breakfast the next morning. This practice is called Time-Restricted Eating. Thus, eating an apple first thing in the morning or a breadstick right before bed would not be the best strategy for weight loss. Eating those things during a shorter eating window (let's say between 10:00am-6:00pm) would encourage weight loss more.

There's more detail on these two concepts in the section "Metabolic Complexity and Sense of Humor" (how often you eat matters / how long you fast matters).

That said, our perspective is that eating only 500-800 calories is already very challenging! *It's not essential for HCG patients to worry about how many times they eat per day or how many hours their eating window is.* However, if one wanted to maximize weight loss, eating on fewer occasions and for fewer hours of the day than the original protocol allows should help.

<u>Under the protein sources listed in the original protocol</u>

Be smart about the category "fresh white fish." That's too broad to be very helpful. Halibut is a fresh white fish that'd be fantastic for HCG Phase 2. Chilean sea bass is a fresh white fish that is oily (and delicious) and terrible for Phase 2. We'll come back to how to make your protein choices in a minute.

Dr. Simeons forbids eating tuna, which is actually a terrific choice for Phase 2, in our opinion. Do avoid what's called "fatty tuna" or *toro* at the sushi bar, though. He also forbids *"...dried, smoked and pickled fish..."* Dried fish like cod are a staple in some cultures. We don't see any reason you couldn't re-constitute dried fish such as *bacalao* while on HCG, as long as it's not an oily fish like mackerel, herring or sardines. In fact, dried cod would be excellent for travel!

Fish that's been smoked is fine, in our opinion, as long as it hasn't been cured in sugar or preserved in oil. For example, some *cold* smoked salmon, like Nova lox or Scottish smoked salmon, are cured in salt and sugar. But there is also *hot* smoked salmon, like Alderwood smoked salmon, which would be fine in small amounts. Hot smoked salmon is fully cooked; it's been smoked over a wood fire, not cured in salt and sugar. In short, any plain, non-oily fish that has been smoked without sugar is a fine way to get more flavor for few additional calories. For example, a little smoked trout could take the place of anchovies in a Caesar salad dressing.

Dr. Simeons allows patients to eat an occasional whole egg, including yolk, if it is combined with the whites of four additional eggs. *We recommend that you eat one whole egg, about once a week, if you would like to, but without those additional egg whites.* That amount of protein in one sitting would likely trigger a larger insulin effect than just eating a whole egg would.

Under vegetables listed in the original protocol

Onions, tomatoes and fennel should be eaten in small amounts, due to their carb count. They taste great (especially together) but many other veggie choices would allow you larger portions.

The Simeons protocol was written in Rome, where fennel, onion and tomato are staples. As always, social context maters! Another example: the Italian palate is quite accustomed to bitter greens. Some of the vegetables on the original protocol, such as chicory and beet greens, reflect this acquired taste.

You needn't be literal about the food lists on the original protocol. Choose HCG-safe foods that you actually like, rather than trying to force an ingredient you don't.

Why Science Supports These Advances

HCG acts mainly upon the hypothalamus to neutralize hunger signals. HCG has other metabolic talents, but it is stellar at neutralizing hunger. Your very low calorie / very low carb intake during Phase 2 is what signals enzymes to begin breaking down your fat for fuel.

Ketosis means that the body gradually shifts from operating on sugar (glycogen) metabolism to operating on your stored fat. This transition takes from a couple of days to a couple of weeks, depending upon your particular enzymes and the amount of stored glycogen in your muscles and liver, primarily. For example, people with Type II Diabetes often have a fatty liver and a fair amount of fat *within* their muscles. Think of a steak that is well-marbled. Each person has to burn through their individual glycogen stores before they get to the fat burning power of ketosis. Thus, a person with Type Ii Diabetes might take longer to get into deep ketosis, but that doesn't mean they've done anything wrong.

While you'll get the most bang for your buck if you stay away from eating fruit, starchy vegetables and crackers while on HCG, eating these foods with special caution will not prevent you from losing weight. If you crush Melba toast to make a crispy coating for baked fish, it does not kill your weight loss project, nor would throwing a few blueberries into your whey protein shake. It's just that you'll want to do as little as possible to interfere with ketosis.

If the crunch of a breadstick is the difference between sticking with the low calorie phase and abandoning it, do it; that's our philosophy. Once you decide to end HCG, you will still have several days of eating very low calories until the hormone is out of your system. It's not as though you can go back to normal food intake right away, so eating something that might slow your weight loss for a day is a better strategy than ending the diet just so you can have a few bites of pasta is. Just think it through with the guidelines we provide you. For example, tossing blackberries rather than blueberries into your whey protein shake is less likely to stall your progress. That's a pretty reasonable adjustment to make.

Dr. Simeons appears to have recommended Melba toast and grissini breadsticks because they contain no oil. That's true, they don't, but neither do many other crackers that are lower in carbohydrate. *Finn Crisp* and *Wasa Thins* for example, would both be a better cracker choice for P2 than grissini or Melba toast would be, because they are much lower in carbohydrate. Two *Finn Crisp* (13 gram serving) have 7 net carbs. Two *Wasa Thins* (17 gram serving) have 8 net carbs. Considering serving size, they are essentially equivalent. In terms of fat, *Finn Crisp* (made of rye) have zero grams and *Wasa Thins* (made of wheat) have 2 grams fat per serving. Both of these crackers offer some crunch, plus the right to feel like a pompous health-food nut.

Finn Crisp crackers are dense and crunchy, with the tang of sourdough and/or caraway. They really taste like something and would be sturdy enough to dip. They wouldn't be great for crumbling as a topping, though. *Wasa Thins* are more neutral in flavor and more delicate in texture, so they'd be good for crumbling to make a topping, but less good for dipping.

We don't actually recommend that you eat crackers on HCG, but we do recommend that you know what will enable you to remain on Phase 2. For some people, the crunch of a cracker is a must-have. If so, choose crackers lower in carbohydrate. That's what *HCG for Foodies* is all about.

Method for Choosing Fruit and Vegetables

Fruits and vegetables are carbohydrates. Since any food high in fat or carbohydrate will interfere with HCG's ability to do its job, we need to be smart about our choices.

Anything high in starch (like the wheat in a breadstick) or sugar (like the pulp of an orange) is capable of returning your body to burning sugar for fuel. This is called being "kicked out of ketosis."

Here are guidelines for your choices of fruits and vegetables while on Phase 2.

Carbohydrate Guidelines

Grams of carbohydrate per 100 grams of fruit or vegetable:
Tier 1 = 0 - 4 carbs   Fine to eat in moderate amounts
Tier 2 = 4.1 - 7 carbs   Fine to eat in smaller amounts
Tier 3 = 7.1 - 9 carbs   Eat a little bit as a special treat
Tier 4 = Over 9 carbs   Not recommended except for flavor

Look up the carbs (per 100 grams) of the fruits and vegetables that interest you. This task will drive you crazy, guaranteed. That's because you will find such inconsistent information: one nutrition database will say that golden beets have 10 g carbs per 100 g, another will say 12 g; yet another source will only have data for purple beets and still another will show golden beets in ounces, not grams. Don't worry about perfection. The point is knowing which fruits and vegetables you can eat on P2 and roughly how much of them you can consume.

Here's the USDA website, which gives the nutritional values of all foods in the same unit of measure that we have used, 100 grams: https://ndb.nal.usda.gov/ndb/

Your choices of foods while on P2 can now be personal and intentional. You'll get some sobering news about foods you like, but you'll also see that there are a great many foods you *can* work into HCG Phase 2.

Our lists of suggested fruits, vegetables and proteins were compiled in the Western United States. This limits our vision. If you are reading this in a different part of the world, you may have access to fruits, vegetables, seafood and meats that we are not familiar with. Use your understanding of local cuisine to enrich our lists of suggested foods!

We cannot possibly imagine all the fruits in Brazil or vegetables in Singapore. We've never seen some of the crustaceans in Australia, fresh fish in the Philippines or the smoked fish in Scandinavia. We don't know all the meats in South Africa, poultry in New Zealand, spices in Jamaica or mustards in Germany. Just think about all the herbs growing in UK gardens and all the berries in Canada! We give you the formula, you do the calculations. While you do that, we'll make travel plans...

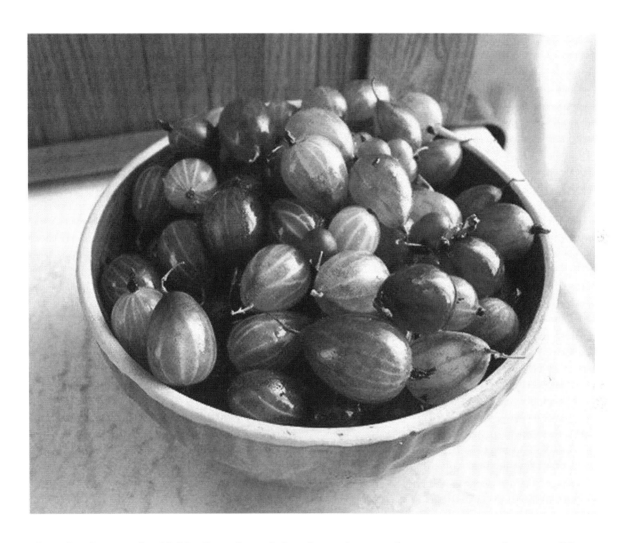

Gooseberries are plentiful in Canada and elsewhere. At 10 carbs per 100 grams, they are a Tier 4 fruit, so you can have a small amount. Perfect for making a sweet-tart relish to serve with meat or fish. Simmer gooseberries with a little water, unflavored gelatin and alternative natural sweetener, like erythritol, stevia or monkfruit extract, until the liquid reduces.

Suggested Fruit Choices

Not an exhaustive list

These carb counts are **per 100 grams**, not per piece of fruit or "per serving." Nutrition data varies by the database you consult, so these numbers jump around a touch, but below are reliable suggestions.

Items on the original Simeons protocol are in bold.

TIER 1 — Moderate amounts ok

None

TIER 2 — Small amounts ok

Rhubarb 4.5g

Lemon 5.4g

Casaba melon 6.6g

Starfruit (carambola) 6.7g

TIER 3 — Only as a treat

Watermelon 7.5g

Strawberry 7.6g

Acerola (West Indian Cherry) 7.7g

Pitanga (Surinam cherry) 7.9g

Grapefruit 7.5 - 9.5g, varies by variety (Florida grapefruit = 7.5g)

Cantaloupe 8.1g

TIER 4 — For flavoring only

Honeydew melon 9g

Lime 9gPrickly pear cactus 9.5g

Peach 9.5g

Pomelo 9.6g

Mulberry 9.8g

Green (unripe) papaya 9.8g

Gooseberry 10.1 g

Nectarine 10.5 g

Asian Pear 10.6 g

Surprisingly poor fruits for HCG

(Grams of carbohydrate per 100 grams fruit)

Apricot 11.1g

Blueberry 12.2g

Pineapple 13g

Navel orange 13g

Fuji apple 15g

Acai berry 15g

Bing cherry 16.2g

Green (unripe) mango 17.5g

When we dip into the nutritional data, there are some intriguing discoveries. Why would casaba melon (6.6 grams) which tastes so sweet, be lower in carbohydrate than blueberries (12.2 grams) which can be tart? People are always yapping about blueberries as a superfood, and blueberries *are* nutritious, but they're not super for losing weight while on HCG.

Why is green, unripe papaya (9.8 grams) okay in small amounts, but green mango (17.5 grams) not okay? Why do limes have nearly twice the carbs of lemons? Ponder such mysteries as your pants get looser.

We hope these details will strengthen your choices on P2. If you make Thai larb, for example, perhaps you'll use a squeeze of lemon juice rather than the traditional lime juice. If you see **shredded green papaya** in the refrigerated section at the Asian market, maybe you'll try a little (it's sour and crunchy) knowing that it's way better for you than a ripe papaya is. If you see a YouTube video with someone putting frozen orange segments in a blender to make sorbet, you'll know that making that same **sorbet out of frozen *grapefruit* segments** with a few drops of stevia would be far safer. Also, it's delicious! Grapefruit is a Tier 3 fruit, with about 7.5 grams carbohydrate per 100 grams. An orange has roughly 12.5 carbs per 100 grams, so it's not on our list of suggested fruits. The more you know, the wiser choices you make, the more weight you lose.

People who practice a low-carb lifestyle sometimes subtract the fiber content from their carb count — they're using *net carbs* when tracking their data. We recommend you make your food choices based on *total carbs* while on HCG.

You can see why some people eat little or no fruit while on Phase 2: very few fruits are low enough in carbohydrate that you could eat very much of them. Fruit is fabulous for creating flavor, though; it's not something you need to omit from your life while on HCG, unless you wish to.

After HCG, we hope you will fall back in love with blueberries and many other plants. Fruits and vegetables offer such exciting taste and texture and they bring amazing phytonutrients to our diet. Lycopene! Flavonoids! Anti-aging effects!

Sound nutritional advice is to "eat the rainbow," meaning eat plants that represent diverse colors, for the phytonutrients they represent and the diversity they bring to our gut microbiome. Imagine what a diet that includes red cabbage, Swiss chard with bright red stalks beneath deep green leaves, orange cauliflower, light green tomatillos, yellow-green avocado, orange bell peppers, white daikon, black cherry tomatoes, purple radicchio, pink grapefruit and red radishes would do for your doo-doo? Imagine peach-colored peaches and plum-colored plums. Perhaps a purple beet from Schrute Farms?

Don't mistake the HCG Diet for real life. There are variables other than carbohydrate count that determine how healthy our food is.

Use fruit to create flavor on HCG

We recommend you *cook with* small amounts of lower-carb fruits, as opposed to eating full portions of higher-carb fruits. This approach plays to foodie strengths; a little fruit can be a clever way to bring a layer of flavor to dishes.

A **spinach salad** with a little pureed strawberry in the vinaigrette is genius, whereas a spinach salad with sliced strawberries is less helpful for your weight loss goal. A plain **whey protein shake** looks and tastes better with a few frozen raspberries tossed in. A slice of chilled, tangy **starfruit** plays well with a hot curry dish. A squeeze of grapefruit improves a **halibut fillet. Pomelo** squeezed into seltzer water tastes a bit like **tonic water.** Slices of **cantaloupe floating in a pitcher of water** will make it taste like you're at the spa. **Stewed rhubarb** tastes great with pork tenderloin. Work your magic.

Suggested Vegetable Choices

Below is a reminder of the carbohydrate tiers we suggest for P2.

Again, we recommend you do eat vegetables, but keep your overall carbohydrate intake during HCG as low as possible, with a maximum of 20 grams total carbs per day.

If you are diabetic, pre-diabetic, have fatty liver, or just know intuitively that you gain weight easily when you eat sugar or starch, you might choose to allow yourself fewer carbs than we suggest here.

Grams of carbohydrate per 100 grams of fruit or vegetable:
Tier 1 = 0 - 4 carbs   **Fine to eat in moderate amounts**
Tier 2 = 4.1 - 7 carbs   **Fine to eat in smaller amounts**
Tier 3 = 7.1 - 9 carbs   **Eat a little bit as a special treat**
Tier 4 = Over 9 carbs   **Not recommended except for flavor**

Here are a few of the vegetables lowest in carbs, thus best for HCG. You take it from here. **Veggies that appeared in the original protocol are in bold.**

TIER 1 — Moderate amounts ok

Watercress 1.3g
Bok choy 1.8g
Bamboo shoots 1.9g
Alfalfa sprouts 2.1g
Cucumber 2.1g
Spinach 2.1 - 2.7g, by variety

Butter lettuce, red lettuce 2.2g

Napa cabbage 2.2g

Radishes 2.6g

Mustard greens, turnip greens 2.8g

Broccoli rabe 2.8g

Yellow crookneck squash, summer squash 2.9g

Celery 3g

Escarole 3g

Zucchini 3.1g

Collard greens 3.2g

Chicory 3.2g

Romaine lettuce 3.3g

Endive 3.3g

Portobello mushroom 3.5g

Mung bean sprouts 3.6g

Cilantro (coriander) 3.7g

Turnip 3.7g

Gai-Lan (Chinese broccoli) 3.8g

Asparagus 3.9g

Chicory 4g

TIER 2 — Small amounts ok

Cherry tomatoes 4.1g

Swiss chard 4.1g

Capers 4.2g

Crimini mushrooms 4.3g

Beet greens 4.3g

Radicchio 4.5g

Chayote squash 4.5g

Green bell pepper 4.6g

Broccoli florets 5g

Green tomatoes 5.1g

White mushrooms 5.3g

Cauliflower 4 - 5.3g, by variety

Cabbage (green, savoy) 5.3g

Pea vines (pea shoots) 5.4g

Kale 5.6g

Thai eggplant 6g

Tomatillo 5.9g [technically a fruit]

Red bell pepper 6g

Kohlrabi 6.2g

Spaghetti squash 6.4g

Jalapeño 6.5g

Shitake mushrooms 6.8g

Chanterelle mushrooms 6.8g

Red cabbage 6.9g

TIER 3 — Only as a treat

Green (string) beans 7g

Scallions (green onions) 7g

Brussels sprouts 7.1g

Canned whole tomatoes 7.3g

Fennel 7.3g

Okra 7.4g

Artichoke 7.75g

Canned pumpkin 8g

Tomato 8g [technically a fruit]

Carrot 8.2g

Chinese long beans 8.4g

Pea pods (sugar snap peas) 8.4g

Rutabaga 8.6g

Jicama 8.8g

TIER 4 — For flavoring purposes only

Yellow onion 9g

Tomato puree or strained tomatoes 9g

Celery root (celeriac) 9.2g

Artichoke hearts 11g

Piquillo peppers 11g

Any other veggie that's 9-11 carbs per 100 grams

Surprisingly poor veggies for HCG

(per 100 grams)

Parsnip 11.4g

Leeks 14g

Shallots 17g

Sunchoke (Jerusalem artichoke) 17g

— Note that white onions have more carbs than yellow onions.

— Note that parsnips have more carbs than carrots.

— Note that leeks have more carbs than scallions.

These are a few examples of the intelligent substitutions possible in P2 cooking. Notice how many veggies are in Tiers 1 and 2 but not on the Simeons protocol!

Garlic (22g carb) is a special case: Though garlic is high carb, you'd never eat 100 grams of it. A little garlic is very useful when you're staring down a bowl of leafy greens as your dinner, though. Our suggestion is this: if you like garlic, use a bit of it to impart flavor. **Roasting garlic and making a paste** gets you sweet, concentrated flavor to work with that you can then dilute. A trick: **infusing a broth** with raw garlic cloves, then removing them, will yield lots of flavor without many carbs.

One medium clove of garlic weighs about three grams, so it's 0.9 carbs. If you use that to flavor a dish that yields two servings, you've got absolutely no problem. What we don't recommend is adding a heaping tablespoon of minced garlic to your stir-fry.

Not surprising, but useful to compare
Russet potato 21.4g
Yuca (cassava) 26.8g
Yam 27.9g

As you may know, potato and cassava (tapioca) starches are common ingredients in gluten-free products. *Being gluten-free is not the same as being low carb.* In order to make something gluten-free, we simply need to avoid the few grains that contain gluten. Other high carb grains and legumes, like rice flour and chickpea flour, are fair game when one is focused on eating gluten free, but are not helpful for HCG.

Don't be bamboozled into buying something gluten-free for use on HCG. Gluten-free products are often *higher* in carbohydrate than their wheat-based counterparts are! Ketosis is facilitated by being *grain free*, not by being gluten free.

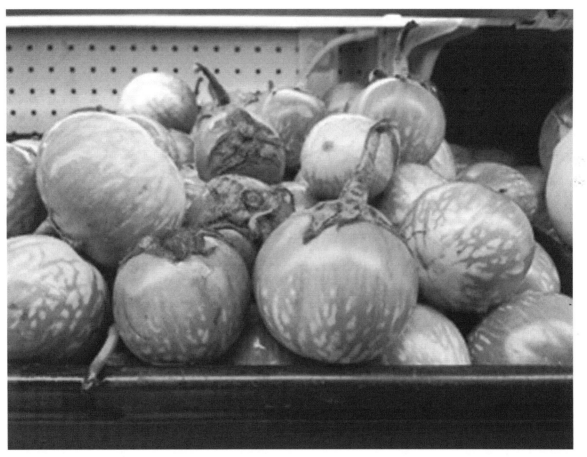

Photo: Dana Falk

Thai eggplant is amazing when cooked on the grill and finished with a drizzle of sherry vinegar. It has only 6g carbs per 100g, so it's a Tier 2 veggie with a lot of potential.

So how many carbs do your favorite veggies have? Do a "Food Search" or a "Nutrient Search" on the USDA website. Here's the tool: https://ndb.nal.usda.gov/ndb/search/list

For a quick and dirty internet search of food content, simply search _____ [food of interest] + nutrition. For example, you could search "nectarine nutrition." That search will give you the stats for nectarines, but you must **use the "amount per" pull-down list to locate 100 grams.** Otherwise, you won't have valid comparisons between the foods you're researching.

Varieties of produce and carbs

Different varieties of the same fruit or vegetable have different carbohydrate content. For example, red cabbage has 7.4 carbs per 100 g but **napa cabbage** has only 3.2 carbs. **Shitake and chanterelle mushrooms** have 6.8 carbs per 100 g but **white button mushrooms** have only 3.3 g! Little **cherry tomatoes** have 10 carbs per 100 g but big old **beefsteak tomatoes** have only 4 carbs. (You've no doubt noticed the difference in sweetness between these two varieties of tomato.)

Researching differences in the carb count for different varieties of the same vegetable is worth your while. As you can see above, you could eat twice as many white button mushrooms as you could shitake mushrooms. We discuss this research process such more under "Twenty Preparations for HCG."

Don't drive yourself crazy with this, but your awareness can be useful. Use the MyFitnessPal app, Carb Manager app, the Noom app, the USDA search tool or Google nutrition searches to increase your awareness. Have five minutes to kill? Look up shallots and onions, which taste similar. Your research makes the decision easy! Shallots have twice the carbs of onions. Choose yellow onion when creating that type of sweet, earthy flavor while on HCG.

The rest of the list is yours to create. For each vegetable that interests you, check the carb content to see whether you could eat a lot, a little or none of this veggie on P2.

A note about the online USDA search tool: you will see the same food listed more than once, with different stats. Try using the word "fresh" or "raw" or "whole" in your description, to narrow your results. Here it is again: https://ndb.nal.usda.gov/ndb/

If the USDA tool drives you crazy, go with the less official but easier internet search for _____ [food] nutrition. For example, Google "cilantro nutrition." Don't forget to use the pull down menu for "amount per" to select 100 grams.

Avoid starchy, high-carb veggies until after Phase 3:

For example, potato, sweet potato, yam, yuca/cassava, taro, lotus root, water chestnut, Jerusalem artichoke, sunchoke, dense flesh (winter) squash like acorn, butternut and kabocha, arrowroot.

Avoid grains like wheat, corn, rice and millet.

Avoid beans and legumes like lentils, soy nuts / edamame / tofu / miso / tempeh or anything called 'vegetable protein,' peanuts, pine nuts, tiger nuts, split peas/green peas, black-eyed peas, chickpeas, black beans, pinto beans, kidney beans, fava beans and lima beans. Finally, a solid excuse not to eat your lima beans.

Until you're done with Phase 3, we suggest your motto for starchy foods be "...*When in doubt, leave it out....*" We want your new weight to stick!

There's much more guidance about maintaining the weight you've lost in the section "Transition to HCG Phase 3."

Method for Choosing Proteins

Protein grams
$$\frac{\text{Protein grams}}{(\text{Fat} + \text{carb})\ \text{grams}}\ \text{per serving} = \text{protein density} = \text{how good for P2}$$
(Fat + carb) grams

The higher this number — the better it is for P2 — the more of it you can eat.

For any protein you're curious about, do the above calculation to see how good it would be while on HCG. Per serving of the food of interest, take # grams protein, divided by # grams (fat + carbohydrate). This gives you that food's "protein density."

Sample Protein Density Calculation

One serving of Argentine Red Shrimp (prawns) from Trader Joe's contains:

38.4 grams of protein

2.4 grams of fat

2.4 grams carbohydrate

The formula is protein ÷ (fat + carbohydrate)

38.4 protein divided by (2.4 fat + 2.4 carb)

= 38.4 divided by 4.8

= 8 is the protein density score for prawns

Any score over 4 is good, so eating prawns would be great for Phase 2.

Our protein density recommendations

* Proteins with a score of four or more (4+) are your best bet.

* Proteins scoring 3-4 are fine in smaller portions.

* **Foods with protein density 2-3 may be used as a minor ingredient**, but should not be the focus of your meal.

Unlike researching safe fruits and vegetables, you don't need to calculate proteins using 100 grams of the food. When selecting proteins, you can apply the formula above using any serving size of the food. Whether you find nutrition data for 1 cup, 3 oz, 100 g or an entire side of beef doesn't matter: just divide the grams protein by grams of (fat + carbs) to find the protein density score.

We are not the only practitioners to advocate for patients making informed decisions about food and portion sizes on HCG rather than blind adherence to the protocol. Anderson & Gustafson (2012), Prinster (2008), LaBoube (2013), Lipman (2018) and others have contributed to this literature. In even greater numbers, of course, are clinicians who teach their patients to make good decisions on the HCG Diet but who have not published these observations.

Suggested Protein Choices

Listed with their protein density score. (Higher is better.)

Not an exhaustive list.

Crawfish tails = 15	Prawns = 8	Canned tuna in water = 20	Canned chicken breast = 13
Calamari = 10.7	Octopus = 4.6	Lobster = 20.6	Crab claw meat = 34
Ahi tuna = 26	Scallops = 4.6	Cherrystone clams = 14.6	Razor clams = 4.5
Halibut = 9.6	Mahi mahi = 21	Trout = 3.6	True cod or ling cod = 21
Yellowtail = 4.4	Dover sole = 8.5	Orange roughy = 23	Red snapper = 17
Bison steak = 8.6	Beef eye round = 4	Beef top round = 3.7	Veal = 7.7
Lamb sirloin = 4.1	Goat = 8.95	Pork tenderloin = 3.8	Venison = 11.2
Egg whites = 12	Thorne vanilla whey protein isolate = 6	TGS unflavored whey protein = 7.7	Turkey breast = 19
Cornish hen white meat = 4.1	Chicken breast = 12.2	Duck breast without skin = 4.6	Turkey leg without skin = 7.8

There are many protein sources that are great for normal life but not good choices for your time on HCG. Beans and legumes, for example, are not on the above list of suggestions because they contain so much starch. (Black beans = .35 protein density!) Yogurt, ricotta, milk, cottage cheese and other fresh "young dairy" are not on the list because they have lactose/natural sugars (skim milk = .72 protein density.) Cheese and other "aged dairy" are not on the list because of their fat content (aged gouda = .88 protein density).

Remember, a protein density score of 3-4 is pretty good. A score over 4 is good; the higher the better.

If you find a dairy or dairy-alternative product that has a reasonable protein density score, you can work it in as a treat on P2. For example, Trader Joe's non-fat cottage cheese = 3.5 protein density. **Trader Joe's 0% Greek yogurt** = 3.1 protein density. If you wanted to make a **tzatziki sauce** out of yogurt + grated cucumber + garlic + salt + lemon juice + mint [optional] that would be fine if you can resist eating a large portion of it and just use it as a dressing or dip.

Remember that all dairy may create weight loss stalls, though. **Goat and sheep milk products** are somewhat less risky than cow milk is, for most people, but it all has the potential to cause a stall. Again, *if it would help you to stick with the low calorie phase*, use a bit of protein-dense dairy. If you've had a little dairy one day, don't be discouraged by any water weight gain you may observe the following day.

Surprisingly poor proteins for HCG

Quinoa = .17
Garden burger = .8
Tempeh = .85
Whole egg = 1.1
Mussels = 1.95
Beef flank steak = 2.5
Chicken thigh without skin = 2.75
Beef liver = 2.9

Fat-free cottage cheese — protein density varies a lot by brand
1.83 (Lucerne)   2.0 (Umpqua)   2.3 (Darigold, Kroeger)
3.5 (Trader Joe's, Clover, Albertson's)

You'll make some discoveries as you research proteins

Isn't it intriguing that turkey dark meat (7.8) is so much better for you than chicken dark meat (2.75) is while on HCG? That ahi tuna (26) can taste so much like yellowtail (4.4) but have so much less fat? That clams (3.6 - 14) are so much safer for P2 than mussels (1.9) are? That goat meat (8.95) tastes like lamb (4.1) but you could eat twice as much of it? That even the leanest, toughest cuts of beef just barely qualify as good choices for Phase 2? (Beef top round = 3.7) That one brand of fat-free cottage cheese would be a really poor choice (Lucerne, 1.83) and another would be okay in small amounts? (Clover, 3.5). Researching ingredients will really pay off for you.

Choose the protein sources that float your boat, but if you are sick of feeling hungry, consider eating some protein you could scarf a huge portion of, like tuna canned in water (22 protein density) or fresh codfish (21 protein density).

On the other hand, if you're hankering for a specific flavor profile — let's say **lemongrass grilled pork tenderloin** (3.8 protein density) — that might be the most satisfying dish you could eat on that day, even though you can't have a lot of it. Your self-awareness is key to whether you choose to eat a lot of something you don't care about or a little of something you're really in the mood for.

Twenty Preparations for HCG

Other than making deliberate food choices, our best advice is that you set aside some time for serious preparation before beginning doses of the hormone. Think of three days as the bare minimum and three weeks as the ideal.

Some of these suggestions are mental preparations — things to think about, anticipate, concentrate on — and some are concrete things for you to do, research or buy. Giving yourself at least three days to prepare before beginning the actual diet will pay off for you big time, in terms of the ease and effectiveness of your HCG experience.

There's more about strategy in the section "Tactics for Changing a Short-Term Behavior." Some of these recommendations are things you could tackle in advance of the diet, so they may help ground your preparations even further.

Concrete Preparations

1. Learn to choose your fruits, vegetables and proteins wisely

Familiarize yourself with the sections of this book that explain how to determine the fruits, vegetables and proteins best for HCG Phase 2. Concentrate on the sections "Method for Choosing Fruits and Vegetables" and "Method for Choosing Proteins." Assure that you're familiar with calculating protein density scores. Know how to determine how many carbs a food has per 100 g. Understand how Tiers 1-4 suggest how much of that food you can eat.

Make a list of the foods and condiments that will help you meet your goals because they taste good to you. *This step will take some time:* you will be looking up the carb count of each individual fruit and vegetable you're curious about, performing calculations on protein sources, making decisions. Investing this energy up front will make the process much less stressful once you're on the hormone and the stakes are high.

If you prefer not to do this research, or you didn't begin reading *HCG for Foodies* until you had begun the diet, just use the list of suggested fruits, vegetables and proteins we have already researched for you; you'll see that there are plenty of options. Once you're rolling on the diet with our suggestions, you can add to these by checking the nutrition data for other foods you discover at the seafood counter, farmer's market and so on.

2. Investigate new ingredients

A great tip for cooking on HCG Phase 2 is to investigate, up-front, which herbs and spices you enjoy. You will be looking for ways to bring flavor to your cooking with very few calories, so having interesting herbs and spices on hand is very helpful. Most of us skip past the chervil and the fenugreek on our way to the basil and the black pepper. Don't do that now — you'll want to know how all kinds of things taste, so you can incorporate them in your HCG cooking. Avoid pre-packaged spice mixes that contain sugar, dextrose or MSG, but from there, the taste tests are up to you.

Part of knowing what you like involves trying things you're unfamiliar with. Do you like thyme but hate rosemary? Try **lemon thyme**; it's awesome. Do you find dill too assertive but want something similar in look with mellow flavor? Try **fennel fronds**, the delicate greens at the top of a fennel bulb. These have a slightly sweet, gentle anise flavor. Do you hate cilantro but want something that's very fresh tasting? Try **celery**

leaves. If you like basil on fresh tomato slices but don't have any in the house, try **fresh tarragon or mint leaves**. Perhaps you can even find pineapple mint or chocolate mint. Want a colorful, earthy spice for your spice rub but don't care for paprika? Try sumac, which is slightly sour and smoky. Set aside time to explore the possibilities online and in your local markets.

You may discover some new favorite ingredients while on HCG if you're willing to explore. At little ethnic markets, health food stores, farmer's markets and outlet grocery stores you'll find veggies, cuts of meat, types of fish, teas, fresh herbs and spice mixes that are new to you. Frankly, even at the most run-of-the-mill grocery store, there are plenty of interesting things we hardly notice.

Korean grocery stores win the prize for best variety of fermented veggies. Read labels when shopping for Korean food, because the delicious Korean chili paste, *gochujang*, has sugar and sesame oil. If you want **kim chee** but don't care for spicy food, you can rinse off the red chili paste or buy the mild cabbage kim chee. Mild kim chee may also be labeled **white kim chee, Napa kim chee or fresh kim chee**. Other fermented foods, like **sauerkraut** and **pickled green tomatoes** are great for your gut health, too, and are safe for P2.

Go forth and find markets you've never been to that are driving distance from your home. Using our stomping grounds near Seattle, Washington as an example, our patients have found a Latino market in Renton, a Russian market in Kent, a Vietnamese market in Factoria, a Persian market in Redmond, an Ethiopian market in SeaTac, an Indian market in Burien and a Filipino market in Tukwila.

Not everyone has access to small ethnic markets, but don't be discouraged. Try this trick if you live somewhere that has mostly mainstream grocery stores: shop at a *different brand name store* than what you usually frequent. Popular grocery chains stock somewhat different products from one another. So if you usually shop at Safeway, Food Lion, H-E-

B, Giant Foods, Kroger/QFC/Fred Meyer/Smith's, Whole Foods, Publix, Sprouts, Shop Rite, Hannaford, Aldi, Hy-Vee, Sam's Club, IGA, Coles, Meijer, Sainsbury's, Walmart, Market Basket, Costco, Harris Teeter, Albertson's, Countdown, Four Square, Sam's Club, Trader Joe's, Costco, Stop & Shop, Jewel, Tesco or some other major market...just try a different grocery store! In some cases, what they have will be substantially different from what you're accustomed to seeing.

This kind of exploration can be really fun, and it's nearly guaranteed to improve your choices while on HCG, but it does take time. If you don't feel like schlepping around town, take to the internet in search of shelf-stable ingredients. Each time you stumble upon a food that intrigues you, enter it into MyFitnessPal, the USDA, Google or some other search to see whether its numbers would work for HCG Phase 2.

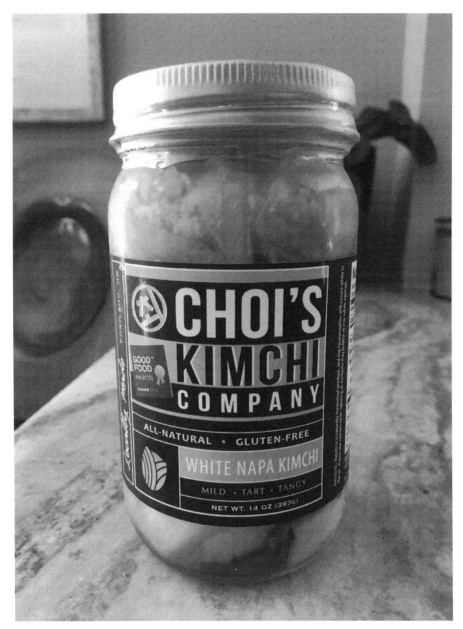

Photo: Dana Falk

Mild kim chee is pretty easy to find, refrigerated, in the produce section at mainstream grocery stores. White kim chee is sour rather than hot. It's fermented, so it's good for your gut microbiome, which facilitates weight loss.

Another way to reduce the effort you expend is to choose a supermarket that's truly super in terms of its selection. Go big. In the Seattle area, for example, Central Market is absolutely top notch for the quality and quantity of their offerings. Natural markets like Whole Foods, New Seasons and Sprouts often have a more narrow selection but a higher proportion of items that would work for HCG. These stores are more likely to carry sugar-free, grain-free and fat-free products as well as products that are non-GMO. Explore whatever is driving distance from your home. For some people, that means five miles. For some foodies, it means 50 miles.

Grocery outlet stores aren't super in their selection, but their prices are irresistible. For example, they often carry big bags of **bite-sized sweet red, yellow and orange bell peppers.** You can pack these for lunch to **scoop tuna salad or bake the world's tiniest meatloaf-stuffed peppers.** You could serve these to company and no one would guess you're eating for HCG.

Look for **minced lemongrass** in the freezer section of Asian markets; it comes in a vacuum-packed bag or a little plastic tub. This is a terrific time saver and is surprisingly inexpensive. Lemongrass makes an awful lot of things taste good.

As you research each food you're considering, you'll see that nutritional information varies by the source you use, which can be frustrating. When you type any food that has no manufacturer's label into MyFitnessPal, for example, there will be multiple offerings. As long as you keep your unit of measure consistent — 100 grams or 1 oz let's say — you'll have valid figures to work with.

We believe it's *well* worth the work to do some exploring for ingredients. One patient told us that she went to a seafood market and never realized how good **fresh red snapper** tastes. Another patient told us that he discovered some tender **choy sum greens** at an Asian market, prepared them with fish sauce and eats them chilled when on HCG. Adding just a few favorite ingredients to your bag of tricks can be a huge help while on Phase 2.

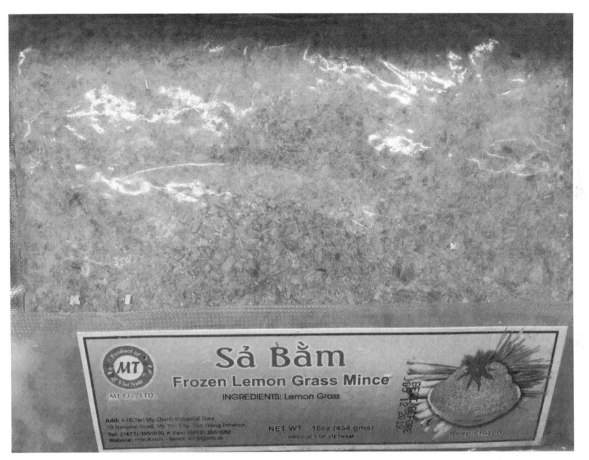

Don't miss minced lemongrass in the freezer section of Southeast Asian markets; it's a serious bargain. Fresh lemongrass tastes fantastic and is worth the work if you just need enough to make a couple of dishes, but it would be expensive and very labor intensive to mince this much fresh lemongrass.

3. Gather supplies

Stock up on ingredients

Do you have **unflavored gelatin** in the house right now? **Unsweetened rice vinegar? Pre-packaged hard boiled eggs? Baby bok choy?** You will have so many more degrees of freedom to prepare what you're in the mood for if you have taken time to gather ingredients in advance.

Having an extra **mini-fridge or freezer** can be a help, as you may stumble upon a great deal that you'd like to buy in bulk. Wholesale stores like Cash and Carry will sometimes stock a humongous bag of deveined prawns, for example. Some veggies last a good long time in the fridge. Consider Brussels sprouts and cabbage for their durability if you're not eager to stock up on produce regularly.

Stock up on food containers, tin foil, plastic zipper bags

Grab yourself a batch of those disposable plastic containers that have tight lids or a full set of glass food storage containers. Upright containers with screw-on lids for your broth and sauces may be especially useful. Dollar stores and grocery outlet stores often carry the off-brand versions of these plastic containers at good prices.

Understandably, some people dislike plastic containers. For this special occasion though, when you're working so hard to create interesting meals with limited calories, there's some beauty in a crappy, lightweight plastic bowl with a lid that you can leave at work, give away or recycle...in other words, not have to wash and not have carry around with you everywhere. You'll be working pretty hard for these few months.

Parchment paper is more useful for HCG than aluminum foil is, because you don't have to grease parchment to keep things from sticking. A silicone mat is useful for baking, as it prevents sticking, but parchment is especially nice because you can wrap up your leftovers and pop them directly in the refrigerator.

Invest in a good bathroom scale

It will probably help boost your motivation to own a digital scale that gives you the smallest increments of weight possible. There are reasonably priced scales that show your weight in increments of 0.2 pounds or 0.1 kilograms. Thus, you'd know if your weight had gone from 286 to 285.8 pounds. You would want to know that, wouldn't you? Better yet, see if you can find a scale that gives you feedback in increments of .1 pounds. That's just one-tenth of a pound, but every little bit of progress is encouraging. A really good scale enables you to see that things are headed in the right direction, even if you haven't lost much in a few days.

It's not necessary for your scale to sync with fitness applications, in our opinion, but it is important that you be getting accurate data on your progress in the smallest weight increments possible. Be certain that the scale you choose can give you an accurate reading at your *starting* weight; scales vary in their capacity. There are a number of companies that make higher capacity bathroom scales and it's easy to find one online that will weigh 550 pounds, for example.

4. Search for and test HCG Recipes

We offer you some great ideas for flavorful and inventive dishes, in our humble opinion, but most of our recipes are pretty loose as compared with a conventional cookbook. A recipe is traditionally written to *remove* the guesswork, to give precise measurements and method. The majority of our recipes actually leave in some of that guesswork, because they are meant to be ideas that people can experiment with and personalize.

Given that many people prefer precise recipes, you may want to spend some of your preparation time looking at HCG recipes in cookbooks and online. These are usually divided into recipes for Phase 2 and Phase 3 of the diet, so be careful not to eat a dish designed for Phase 3 while you're doing the very low fat, very low calorie Phase 2.

Once you have found recipes that intrigue you, pretend you're on *America's Test Kitchen* and try actually making them. Not everyone invests the time it takes to test dishes before they are on the HCG hormone, but you will be happy with yourself if you do this. As you know, it's common for recipes to turn out tasting different from what we'd imagined — sometimes better, sometimes worse.

5. Cook in bulk and freeze your favorites

If you stumble upon a recipe you like, make a bunch of it. That's a particularly good plan if you've found a dish that requires time and effort. Put several extra servings in the fridge and the rest of it in the freezer, all portioned out; you'll be so happy you did. Right now you are sick of the hot and sour soup with Chinese meatballs you made, but it will taste amazing a week from now when you need a quick dinner. Having that frozen soup on hand may keep you from grabbing something that doesn't meet your goals.

Cooking in bulk is an aspect of your preparation you could embark on a month or so before you begin HCG. Not only does having the food prepared make the diet easier when the time comes, it also forces you to practice making HCG meals. How much broth do you put in a "stir fry" when you can't use oil? Is there a way to make a zucchini lasagne that doesn't become watery? Can you find a dish you like that's made with shirataki noodles? How much mushroom do you need to put in a turkey meatloaf to keep it from drying out? Is there a salad dressing you like enough that it would encourage you to eat salad? Conduct trial runs.

6. You don't have to cook

Hey look, not everyone cares about how creative or flavorful their meals are. Some other people do care, but they don't have time to fuss with making artisan **lobster broth so their leafy greens will taste good.** Even foodies like to keep it simple sometimes. So it's worth saying here, when we're discussing preparation for the diet — if you don't want to cook while you're on HCG, you don't actually have to.

Good salad bars these days offer things like fresh spinach, raw broccoli, steamed cauliflower, white meat chicken. There are chilled radish slices, shredded zucchini, shredded cabbage. Sliced bell peppers. Chopped celery. Baked cod. Whole, hard-boiled eggs. Mixed baby greens. Cold, sliced chicken breast. Kale salad and cole slaw made without the dressings.

Individual bags of hard boiled eggs are sold near the fresh eggs and Costco sells a huge box of hard boiled egg two-packs. You can **buy a bag of lettuce and dump a can of tuna on it.** You can find **sashimi in the grab n' go section** of many markets. **Roasted turkey breast** (not turkey lunch meat) is sold by the pound at some grocery store delis. **Plain, cooked baby shrimp and prawns** are often available under plastic wrap in the seafood section. **Colorful mini bell peppers** come in a zip top bag. **Fresh crab meat comes canned**, and it's pretty darn good. Little **Persian cucumbers and pickling cucumbers** are sturdy; you can tote them around without making a mess.

We are delighted to offer ideas for creating flavorful food, but it's entirely possible to make it through P2 without bothering with all of that. You may want to use your preparation time to familiarize yourself with inviting grab n' go options at local stores and restaurant takeout rather than exploring new ingredients. For example, buying **smoked chicken by the pound at a barbecue place** and requesting "sauce on the side," would taste great on a salad. Obviously you wouldn't choose pulled pork butt, fatty beef brisket or hot links at a barbecue place, but smoked chicken? That smoke is a lot of extra flavor for no additional calories. Mediterranean and Middle Eastern restaurants may have a chicken shwarma salad on the menu. Get the dressing on the side and you have a flavorful meal with no cooking.

If all these ideas for cooking overwhelm you, ignore everything except our lists of Suggested Choices for fruit, vegetables and proteins. Buy your favorite items on these three lists of safe foods and eat them for your time on HCG Phase 2.

7. Begin taking MCT oil in advance

One of the supplies you will probably buy is a high quality MCT oil. This is a supplement that's helpful for getting into ketosis, so it facilitates weight loss while on HCG. MCT oil has its own section later in the book; worth reading now if you choose to build slowly.

You'll be allowed 2-3 tablespoons of MCT oil per day while you're on the HCG Diet, and it's the *only* oil you will have access to, so it's really valuable to your cooking. You can use it to make pesto, vinaigrette and other salad dressings, creamy hot beverages and more. Because MCT oil assists ketosis, it also assists with reducing your appetite. In short, it's a big help.

Here's the catch: your tummy will probably not be able to tolerate 2-3 tablespoons of MCT oil right away. Most people experience diarrhea, cramps or nausea when they introduce MCT oil for the first time, unless they begin with a small amount and build slowly from there. It's a lot of free fatty acids for your digestive tract to manage.

We think a valuable preparation for your round of HCG would be to begin building your tolerance for MCT oil in advance, one-half teaspoon at a time. Ideally, you should be able to comfortably digest all three tablespoons (taken half in the morning, half in the evening) by the time you begin the very low calorie phase of the diet. This way, by the time you need that 2-3 tablespoons as an aid to fat burning and appetite control, you will actually be able to consume the full dose.

If preparing your digestive system for MCT oil 1/2 teaspoon at a time is the goal, the math would look like this:

— 3 tablespoons = 9 teaspoons
— Begin with 1/2 teaspoon of MCT oil and increase your intake by 1/2 teaspoon each day.
— It will take 18 days to reach the full, three tablespoon dose.
— *Thus you'd need to start MCT oil 18 days prior to the Loading Phase of the diet.*

If you don't have that kind of lead time as you're reading this, just remember to build your MCT dose gradually, slowing the pace if you experience explosive diarrhea; that's pretty straightforward math.

8. Test food sensitivities in advance

If you really, truly want the best possible results on HCG, this suggestion will be worthwhile preparation. Testing for food sensitivities before HCG is work that yields valuable information.

When you're on the hormone, eating something you have a slight food intolerance to (even a food that's fine for HCG) could make the scale go up temporarily, due to water retention. Eating that food could stall your weight loss. This is because when our body prefers we not eat something, and we do, it responds with inflammation. This can be extremely discouraging, especially since you didn't do anything wrong!

Let's say you found out through testing that you have a sensitivity to strawberries — not an allergy, just a food intolerance. You could easily avoid strawberries while on HCG, even though they are technically something people eat on Phase 2. Perhaps you would decide upon raspberries instead, just to prevent weight stalls. That would be useful information to have about your body, wouldn't it?

There are a variety of ways to gather information about food sensitivities; each of these has its supporters and its critics. In brief, there are in-clinic blood draws, scratch tests, an electro-dermal test (Q Scan) or consultation with a healthcare provider who could guide you through an elimination diet. At home, you might purchase a food sensitivity kit online that you mail in for results or you may conduct your own elimination diet.

The independent elimination diet is what we describe in a later section of the book, called "Guide to Testing Food Sensitivities." For more conclusive results prior to HCG, though, we suggest you look into blood work or an electro-dermal test with a healthcare professional.

9. Test your response to alternative natural sweeteners

Skip ahead to the section "Alternative Natural Sweeteners." There's a discussion there of your safe choices while on HCG. These are not sugars, like maple syrup and they're not artificial sweeteners, like aspartame. They are *alternative natural sweeteners*, like stevia.

There is disagreement about whether patients should be encouraged to use alternative natural sweeteners while on HCG. For some people, sweeteners of any kind will keep cravings alive. For others, a tiny bit of sweetness is what enables them to stick with the low calorie diet. So our advice is this: jump ahead to the section "Alternative Natural Sweeteners." Read it and decide whether or not you want to try alternative natural sweeteners.

If you do decide to use alternative natural sweeteners like stevia, erythritol, xylitol, allulose or monk fruit, prepare for HCG by sampling a variety of them. Finding the brand(s) that work well for your digestive system, in advance, would be time well-spent.

People vary by which sweetener they prefer in taste and especially by which cause them gastrointestinal problems like heartburn, gas or diarrhea. Let's say you do a 30 day round of HCG; you might not want the first ten days of that to be ordering and experimenting with sweeteners. It's best not to be hungry *and* gassy.

10. Take your measurements

This may seem like an unsavory task, but later on, you'll be very pleased you did this before you began the diet. The rationale for this task is described in preparation tip #19, "Learn the Science of Clinical Obesity." Spoiler alert: sometimes you will get smaller but not lighter. It's important you be able to see that progress.

The more measurements you take, the more opportunities you'll have to observe change. Don't stop with chest and waist. Measure several places on your chest and rib cage, several places on your tummy, hips and tush. Measure your calves and ankles, not just your thighs. Measure your forearm and wrists, not just your upper arm. Perhaps your neck, even the circumference of your face. That may sound strange, but our faces get less round when we lose weight, right?

Even if you feel like avoiding measurements, it's important you do it (and do it early). In just the first week of HCG you will probably lose enough fat that some of these measurements will change. Let's capture that accomplishment.

Mental Preparations

11. "Giving it a shot" vs. really committing

Sometimes we undertake a change half-heartedly. It's not laziness, it's just that we don't fully expect to succeed. It can be a relief to tell ourselves *"...At least I gave it a shot...."*

This is an unconscious process, not a mindful plan to be half-hearted. Telling yourself that you "tried everything" is easier than making a big change is. Prepare for HCG by doing some self-reflection. Are you just giving HCG a whirl or are you really going at it full force?

Of course, there are times we realize from the start that we won't make big sacrifices for a project, but typically we're more optimistic (and less insightful) than that. Even if we've tried to master a project several times and have always half-assed it, we don't necessarily realize that the reason we stumbled is that we didn't try hard enough. We want to learn French but are not willing to take a class, want to write a novel but are not willing to carve out the time, want to build muscle but are not willing to be sore the next day, want to do oil painting but don't want to mess up a room.

When an actor really pulls out the stops, we say he or she committed in that role. They were willing to look silly or ugly or vulnerable or unlikeable in some way, because they knew it wouldn't be a compelling performance unless they did. This same principle applies to major life changes like losing weight: you can "give it a shot" or you can really commit.

Choosing to fully commit to your health is more vulnerable than exerting minimal effort is. Actually trying your best means you have the potential to disappoint yourself, to see what you are truly capable of. We use procrastination all the time to protect ourselves in this way. In school, if you wrote a big paper the night before, and got a B, you'd never know what grade you'd have gotten if you'd worked on it longer. Maybe you'd have gotten an A, but maybe the truth is that you're a 'B' writer. You won't know which it is, because you wrote it the night before. Less effort feels safe, emotionally.

See if you can pull out the stops on this round of HCG. You can prepare for this commitment: *make a list of the things you have not changed with past attempts at goals:*

— Have you kept your goal a secret, when telling people honestly what you're working on would have been more practical?

— Have you told yourself you would keep data on your progress, but abandoned the work of tracking those details?

— Have you told yourself you would set time aside each day for some practice, like meditation, lifting weights or organizing, but not actually carved out the time to do so?

— Have you told yourself you'd spend whatever money it takes to increase your chances of success with some goal, but used those expenses as a reason you meandered off course?

Take an honest inventory of what you did *not* change when you were "giving it a shot." Now see how specific you can get about what you would need to change if you decided to really commit on your round of HCG.

12. Shuffle priorities

During periods of transition we often re-arrange our priorities, intentionally or unintentionally. In fact, we often first *notice* that we're in transition because we can feel how a situation has demanded we do things differently than we would ordinarily.

Adaptability is key to shifting your priorities. Your usual style may not be useful when trying to make an important change. For example, many people place a high value on saving money, but need to spend more when something important lies in the balance. Some people crave time with other people, but need to prioritize time alone when working hard on a project. Some people do not value a focus on physical appearance, but need to spend some time on their looks for a bit without feeling like a sellout. Some people place a high value on efficiency, but need to do things slowly and carefully while on HCG.

A shift of attention may be temporary, like missing work to care for someone recovering from surgery, or it may be a change in priorities for the foreseeable future, like taking better care of your blood pressure because you now have children. For foodies, letting go of the need for meals to always be delicious can be a meaningful, long-term shift of priorities.

The ability to shuffle one's priorities based on some changing reality is a sign of psychological resilience. Adaptability is often much more of a strength than sticking to your guns is. Surely you've noticed there are people who cannot change their mind and pivot as new information becomes available. In fact, in some circles, being flexible is considered weak and being stubborn is considered strong! People who think of adaptability as a weakness are prone to emotional outbursts such as shutting down, being irritable or being highly critical of others. (Did you realize that shutting down when overwhelmed is a kind of emotional outburst?) In Psychology, this is called being "brittle."

If you live or work in an environment that treats flexibility as a weakness, give this some thought as you prepare for HCG. Look hard at what you may need to set aside for a month or two if you want to lose as much as possible while on the hormone.

We will prattle on for many pages about how to be inventive when you have fewer ingredients to work with, but the truth is, taste does not need to be your priority right now unless you want it to be. If you can be satisfied with 'good enough' for now and ease your high standards, that adaptability will serve you well. Perhaps your highest priority right now is to maximize your round of HCG.

13. Check your desire to rebel

Sometimes when we approach a change, we kick into rebellion without even realizing it. Part of your preparation for a round of HCG might be to examine whether you are pushing back against the project in any way. Resisting any preparation for the diet might actually be a way to tell that you're pushing back.

As you prepare mentally for the HCG diet, reflect on your past attempts. Have you sabotaged or avoided sustained weight loss in the past because someone implied that you *should* diet? Are you a woman who believes that taking action on weight loss would be selling-out feminist values? Are you a man who thinks dieting is not masculine enough? Do you think that dieting suggests low self esteem? Have you resented denying yourself the foods you love and begun to drift away from taking it seriously? If so, catch yourself in the preparation stage, before you can sabotage your own work.

Sigmund Freud wrote about unconscious rebellion in The Psychopathology of Everyday Life (1901), *"...I was under a constraint to which I had not entirely resigned myself, so I showed my protest by forgetting...."* In other words, Freud realized that he had not been following through with something because he felt trapped by expectations.

We all drag our feet at times. We're passive because someone asked us to make a change, rather than it being our own goal. We rebel with inaction. We don't complete something we thought was a priority. Even people who aren't rebellious by nature do this without realizing it.

Any time you bring an unconscious thought into conscious awareness, it exerts less power over your mood and behavior. Turning unconscious beliefs into conscious thoughts is the goal of some kinds of therapy, in fact. You can prepare for your round of HCG by reflecting on how you tend to rebel and by catching those signs early.

14. Factor-in social expectations

The ability to gracefully manage social expectations will in large part determine your success on HCG; it's obviously an important part of your preparation for the diet. We offer some suggestions below, but only you know what your own support system and challenges look like. You may be able to design some additional strategies for the social expectations you personally will face.

Lay low for awhile

Choose a time frame for HCG during which you have few social commitments. Some people decide that they will not initiate any get-togethers while on HCG, but will accept an invitation from someone who would be supportive. Other people push all invitations back on the calendar until they have made it one week into Phase 3, when they will be able to eat a little fat and a reasonable enough number of calories that they could eat out.

If you decide to get together with someone you believe will be supportive while you're on Phase 2, they have got to be such cool people that you could say, "…I'm gonna bring some of my own food. Hope you don't mind…" and they would be on board. Bring something you could easily share, like meatballs, chicken kebabs, or crab and cucumber sushi rolls.

Think about restaurants that work for P2

Even if you have done a good job of keeping your calendar clear, it's likely you'll have to eat out at some point while on HCG. One strategy is to think in advance of restaurants or types of cuisine that would enable you to stay on plan.

For example, at places like **Chipotle** and **Qdoba**, where you choose what goes on your taco salad, you might order **grilled, spiced chicken breast on salad greens**. At Japanese restaurants that have sushi you can order **sashimi**. Some teriyaki joints offer **char-broiled chicken breast** (it's typically chicken *thigh* when you order regular teriyaki). If they grill chicken breast and give you sauce on the side, you're perfect. You could choose a restaurant or grocery store that's known for having a great salad bar. At an **oyster bar** you could probably find shrimp, crab and clams as well, if you don't care for raw oysters.

At a barbecue place that offers **smoked chicken**, you can go for the breast and remove the skin. Their **collard greens** may have been cooked with a ham hock, but ask! Steak houses almost always have a **side of asparagus** (hold the butter) and some fresh fish on the menu. Mediterranean restaurants often have grilled fish (ask for no olive oil) or meat kebabs (get whole chunks of chicken, not gyro meat). Seafood restaurants don't love serving you **mahi mahi without the sauce**, but will usually do it. Tip well.

Easier and more fun than going out to eat when on Phase 2 is having a picnic, as weather allows. You have so much more control this way. Bring enough P2 food to share...**fresh turkey breast with HCG cranberry sauce, homemade cole slaw, a few beautiful slices of star fruit or chilled casaba melon, a Bai peach iced tea or Hint water watermelon flavor.**

Put your best dish forward

If you will be eating with other people, whether at a restaurant, in a private home or in the great outdoors, this is the time to bring along your very best P2 grub. Bring your **homemade turkey-garlic meatballs with HCG barbecue sauce**, not canned tuna and celery sticks. Bring your **chicken breast or pork tenderloin rolled with pesto and cut into pinwheels**, or your **ahi tuna sushi roll with cauliflower rice and wasabi**, not a dry spinach salad.

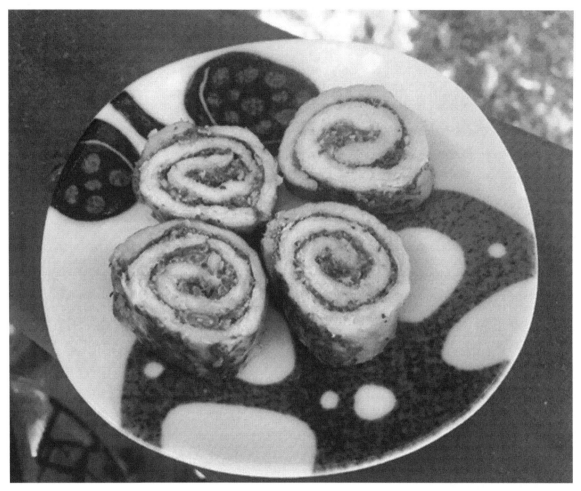

Photo: Dana Falk

What fool would tease you about eating this? Pork tenderloin is pounded thin, spread with spinach-basil MCT pesto, rolled up and baked to an internal temp of 160° F. Let cool, so pesto won't ooze out, then slice into pinwheels. What is pictured is only 60 grams of meat. If you your day allowed for 90 grams of pork tenderloin, for example, you could have six of these pinwheels rather than four.

It's never wise to assume there will be food you can eat when you're going when you're on HCG Phase 2. If you don't want to call attention to your eating or worry people who may think you're on a crash diet, make the food you bring delicious enough to share.

If you're not inclined to cook, you can buy something you will eat that others would enjoy: **fresh strawberries, cold prawns, multi-colored mini bell peppers, crab legs, mini meatloafs baked in silicone molds, green tea gelatin squares.**

What if you're going to a larger event and don't want to treat 20 people to crab legs? How about bringing **brined chicken breasts, dressed baby arugula salad** and hamburger buns? Grill the chicken. Everyone else has the choice of eating the grilled chicken as a sandwich or as a salad. You will choose the salad, of course. Pro Tip: Don't bring delicious brioche buns that you will actually want! Bring pale, crappy supermarket hamburger buns. The people eating a free chicken sandwich with arugula can cope with having it on an ordinary bun.

Putting forth some tasty food calls less attention to your diet. No one will feel sorry for you or think you're on a "crash diet" if you're eating **pork larb with lime juice in lettuce cups.**

Find the right words

Often it helps to rehearse what you will say when people inquire about why you're eating small portions, why you're losing weight, why you decline their freshly baked muffins. It may seem goofy to "prepare a statement" about why you're eating carefully for several weeks, but having your talking points in place can be very useful.

It's important you craft something that's in your voice, that conveys whatever is a natural tone for you. That tone may be to dodge the question, to be warm and explain fully, to answer with a partial truth, to be irritable so people will back off...so many options!

Remember that it's entirely possible to answer questions gently but with a tone that communicates *"...This is private; that's all I'd like to say...."* Whatever your choice, we do recommend literally planning what you'll say.

Here are some possible styles, to get you started:

— Some people phrase a statement **directly and optimistically**, like this: "...I know it may look unusual, but this is something special I'm doing for myself, and I'm doing it with the help of a _____ (healthcare professional). It's a project I've been looking forward to and I think it's a great opportunity...."

— Some people approach social expectations by **front-loading an explanation**: "...I may not be super fun to have as a guest today. I'm eating very carefully for the next few weeks to address my insulin and glucose issues. I knew you'd understand but just wanted to share that with you...." You'd probably use this approach only with people you are fond of.

— Some people increase their closeness with friends when they begin the diet by giving them thorough **enough information to be really supportive**. They might say, "... When we get together for movies, if I bring turkey wraps for us both, would you have some?..." They might also say, "...I can't have the ranch dip right now, but would you cut up extra bell peppers for me? They're my favorite...."

— Some people decide to **fib a little** and say, "...I'm on an elimination diet right now, trying to figure out what foods I'm allergic to...." That's a partial truth: you *are* on an elimination diet. When you get to Phase 3 of your HCG round, you may choose to re-introduce foods one at a time, which will yield information about your food sensitivities.

— Some people make light of what they're doing as a way of **changing the subject**. They might say, "...Everyone has their special dietary needs these days, right? You've got people who don't drink, who won't eat meat, or nuts, or bread; it's crazy. I'm leaving out some things right now, too...."

As long as you are willing to do whatever it takes to eat thoughtfully while you're on HCG, address social expectations any way you choose. We hear from *so* many patients that they were able to keep with their plan, except while eating with other people. They say they felt embarrassed about needing something different. They didn't want to ruin the spirit of the event, didn't want to be "rude" by turning down homemade food, didn't want to seem like they were on a diet of any kind. Essentially, people tell us that they work very successfully at eating Phase 2 foods when at home, but get discombobulated when facing social situations.

You could potentially lose several days worth of diet effort this way. It wouldn't be because you were too hungry, or hadn't shopped for ingredients, or hadn't prepared meals or didn't track your eating. You would backslide simply because they were too chicken to take care of business with other people around. You'll need to work *extra hard* in social situations; you can do it.

You needn't over-share if you don't want to, just prepare a little something to say. Most friends and family kind of admire someone who is taking action on their health issues, but it's certainly possible someone will be critical of your efforts. Aren't those the people who are *always* critical of others, though?

Prepare by thinking of a few ways to say that you realize you are eating differently at the moment but that *it's what you want to do*. Your choice of words is important.

Declining food

For interactions in which you wouldn't normally discuss your health with the other person, you can decline some food they offer by simply saying, "…Oh thank you, not right now…" rather than "…I can't eat that, because _____."

Also very effective is saying, "…No thanks, I'm not a big fan of _____." They may express surprise that you "don't like popcorn," but they probably won't pursue it. We all know a few people who don't care for milk chocolate, soda pop, pizza, red wine, buffalo wings, vanilla lattes or bagels. What do all these foods have in common? They are notorious for causing heartburn. That could be the reason you're "not a big fan."

Foods with sugar, starch, carbonation, tomato, tannins and spices are often painful for people with acid reflux. If a friend pushes back on why you "don't like red wine," you might tell them that it gives you acid stomach, that it causes migraines, or just say, "…I like red wine more than it likes me…." This is a true statement for many people.

We discuss much more about how to deal with social expectations and difficult people while on HCG in the "Interpersonal Skills for Transitions" section.

15. Consider expensive foods

You know how some people love **lobster and crab**, but never buy them because they are so expensive? During Phase 2, you might prepare your budget for some pricey foods. If these items are really delicious to you, they may be worth the expense.

The thing is, P2 is really hard, but it's time-limited. These two expensive foods, lobster and crab, are great examples of absolutely fantastic protein choices for HCG. Costco sells lobster tails in 4-packs and whole crabs in 3-packs. **Save the shells to make broth; it will make leafy greens taste much better.** Costco also sells king crab legs that are so luscious you'll devour them in the parking lot. These are expensive, special occasion purchases and this is a special occasion.

Look for other foods you might not ordinarily splurge on but might make you happy now: **White asparagus. Halibut cheeks. Chanterelle mushrooms. Smoked maldon sea salt. Heirloom tomatoes. Saffron. Squash blossoms. Grass-fed veal.** You get the picture.

16. You don't have to prioritize flavor

As you do your mental preparation for the HCG diet, consider the possibility of purposely keeping things dull, if you think this would be a good exercise for you personally. Understanding good flavor and how to create it is a talent that can easily tumble into food obsession. If you wish to, use Phase 2 as a time to practice reducing your need for food to always be special and delicious. Experiment with tuning down that part of your personality.

Strangely, many people have a non-compulsive relationship with food. (It's quite bewildering, isn't it?) These people don't really care about the ritual of reading about, shopping for, traveling for, cooking, reviewing or eating food, they just need a way to address hunger. Play around the edges of this attitude for the month or so you are on HCG and see if you can re-frame deliciousness as a special occasion rather than a necessity. There's a practical section at the end of the book called "How to Overcome Compulsive Eating."

If you keep a journal, how often you think about food would be an interesting topic to write about. Do you get more work done when you free up some bandwidth that was devoted to food? Do you enjoy trying on the identity of someone who doesn't think much about food unless they are hungry? Do you find you have more tolerance for food that's "okay but not great" than you thought you did?

If you are experimenting with not prioritizing food that's special, you will free up some time and energy. For example, instead of **slow cooking on-the-bone chicken** breast in broth and tarragon for five hours to impart flavor, you could just plop some **skinless chicken tenders into salted boiling water**, drain them, toss them in a zipper bag and head off to work. It would be very bland, but it's perfectly fine and it's strategic: it saves you time, meets your nutritional goals for Phase 2 and helps you to experiment with more independence from food. It's a quick n' dirty workday lunch that accomplishes several goals.

17. Accept potential waste

HCG will be easier if you temporarily relax concerns about food waste. This is an unusual 23-43 days of your life that will depart from your normal practices. For example, when you are zealously trimming all the fat from a chicken breast, you will lose more of that meat than usual. If that bugs you, freeze the fat with meat attached and cook with that tasty chicken schmalz a few weeks after you're done taking the hormone.

Some foods may not stay fresh as long as it takes to finish them when you're eating such small portions. Also, some foods don't taste good after they've been frozen. If you want to minimize waste, freeze what you can, but know it's possible you'll waste some food. You will also be using far more egg whites than egg yolks for a time. If you're concerned about wasting them, give the yolks to someone who can make quiche, custard or ice cream. You might also **hard boil your eggs**, eat the whites towards the end of Phase 2 and save the yolks until you're in Phase 3.

In general, prepare mentally for a little more waste than is characteristic of you; it's a means to an end.

18. Learn how your efforts make HCG work

A behind-the-scenes view of what your body is doing on HCG can be tremendously helpful. You'll have a lot of decisions to make and a lot of rules to follow. Knowing *why* you're following these instructions makes it feel more rational, less arbitrary. The basics: the hormone you'll be taking is excellent at mobilizing the fat that your body has stored. Normally, you burn glucose for energy, but when on HCG, you'll be burning fat. With fat being mobilized in this way, you'll feel less hungry than you would ordinarily. This is what makes it possible to eat so few calories.

Specifically, here is how your efforts make HCG work:

The reason you have to be so hyper about calories on HCG:
Unless you consume fewer calories than your body needs, it will have no reason to pull from your fat stores.

The reason you have to be so hyper about eating very little fat on HCG:
Your body will always utilize the fat you're *feeding* it before it would turn to the fat you have stored. Any dietary fat you eat while on HCG would have come off your body, but doesn't.

The reason you have to be so hyper about carbs on HCG:
Once inside your system, all carbs raise your blood sugar. Sugars encourage your body to burn glucose for fuel, instead of fat. When you eat carbs while on HCG, your body receives a mixed message. You have given it a hormone that asks it to *burn* fat, then eaten foods that instruct it to *store* fat. The more carbohydrate you eat while on HCG, the more confused your body will become about what you want it to do.

These three principles should make absolute sense to you as you embark on HCG. Most questions anyone would ask you trace back to these points. Also, any time you have a crisis of faith about why you're tracking every bite you take, you can come back to your understanding about how your efforts matter.

Spot the science of clinical obesity

This is #19 on the list of preparations, but it deserves special attention. You may notice that we explain the science of obesity more than once in this book. That's because most people think they know what keeps people overweight, but they don't. Most people don't know, for example, that there are different kinds of fat cells. We hope that as part of your preparation for the diet, you will get familiar with obesity as a chronic illness, not just as a social phenomenon. We think that having this background will be useful for you while on the diet if you have been overweight for a while, even if you have never been obese.

Here's the science: people who have been overweight for a long time have the kind of fat cells that like to stick around. By maintaining a higher weight over time, we've actually told the fat cells to stick around, which has created a relatively high "set point" for us.

It feels unfair, but people who are average weight to slightly overweight have an easier time burning fat than people who have more to lose. When a person's set point is lower, their body isn't resisting the process. If you have been overweight more often than not, your body needs reassurance that losing weight is what you really want it to do...so it drops two pounds, then bounces back up one pound.

Think of it this way: it's like asking someone who has lived in Florida for many years if they are certain — really certain — that they want to move to Alaska. They would have to buy a lot of thermal underwear and fur-lined boots before their plan to move from hot weather to cold would seem convincing. This is what your endocrine system is puzzling over when you've been overweight most of your life and are now asking it make your body's set point lower. Are you *sure* you don't want more tank tops? That is what you've always worn.

Just as there are different kinds of fat *cells*, there are different types of fat *stores*. Visceral fat stores are quite different from the subcutaneous fat just beneath your skin. Visceral fat lives in and around the organs of the abdomen, *behind* your abdomen wall; you can't "pinch an inch" of visceral fat. Visceral fat is associated with patients having more difficulty losing weight. Why? Because visceral fat isn't just for storage; it acts like an endocrine organ, secreting chemicals called inflammatory mediators. In short, it ain't good.

The fat just beneath our skin makes fitting into old clothes frustrating, but it doesn't make it harder for us to lose weight. Having visceral fat, for example having a fatty liver, *that is* frustrating.

The bridge between having visceral fat and having a tough time losing weight is insulin resistance. A person with insulin resistance has been over-producing the insulin hormone for so long, the body begins to ignore it. It's essentially a case of "The Boy Who Cried Wolf." Insulin resistance is one of the most common reasons people have special difficulty losing weight.

To review: chronically overweight people have a type of fat store that makes it difficult for them to lose fat stores! *One rationale for a low calorie, ketogenic diet with HCG is that it's one of the few ways to address visceral fat.* In other words, HCG works on a lot of levels.

Re-read the above paragraph if you have smart alecks in your life who think that weight loss is simply about caloric intake or that HCG is a fad diet. There's something more complex at play than what you eat, especially for people who have been overweight much of their lives.

If you might have been tempted to judge your success based only upon how many pounds you lose, you now understand how that's short-sighted: losing visceral fat is far more important than losing subcutaneous fat is. Why? Because it is more relevant to your long term ability to keep weight off. Visceral fat loss may or may not be visible on the scale.

If you go from having a fatty liver to being in the healthy range for visceral fat while on HCG, that's a huge slam dunk. The loss of fat in and around your liver will make it easier for you to lose weight across your lifetime. Lower visceral fat means minimizing hyperinsulinemia (over-production of insulin). When your body isn't over-producing the hormone that tells it to store fat, your body actually hears when you tell it to lose weight. With more visceral fat, your weight loss efforts may fall on deaf ears.

There are body composition analyses that can measure your progress with visceral fat. The Bio-Impedance Analysis (BIA) and the DEXA Scan both provide this information. If this testing is available to you, it's very helpful to look at your visceral fat periodically during your round of HCG, the same way you would pay attention to how your clothes are fitting.

*Patient is on HCG Week 3. Look at the right side, **Visceral Fat Level**. His/her fatty liver is now in the normal range, 10. Three weeks ago, it was 14 (quite unhealthy). Visceral fat creates long-term weight loss resistance. Losing a fatty liver is bigger news than losing weight is.*

20. The intensity is temporary

Prepare yourself mentally for how hard this diet is and how great the rewards are. That combination is intense, but it's temporary. The way you will eat on HCG Phase 2 isn't sustainable and it isn't meant to be. You would not be eating so few calories and so little fat in real life. In fact, once you're off the hormone treatment, this would not even be an effective way to lose weight. With so few calories, you would lower your metabolism. With so little healthy fat, you would rarely feel satisfied.

HCG Phase 2 is a special, short-term project. Think of this project the way you did Finals Week in school: you'll work your ass off for a short time, making sacrifices you wouldn't ordinarily make, because doing so right now is likely to be rewarding. Afterwards, you'll still need to study to do well, but you won't need to pull all-nighters.

Doing HCG skillfully requires a level of nit-picky concentration that is out of character for many people. Prepare yourself mentally for the hard work of researching ingredients, preparing special meals and tracking your caloric intake, but remember that the emotional intensity of this project is time-limited.

Guidelines for the Loading Phase

Phase 1 of the HCG Diet is those few days prior to the start of the very low calorie period and is usually referred to as the Loading Phase. At this time, you'll be taking the HCG hormone but will be eating *high* fat instead of low fat — very high fat. This is because you're trying to put your body into ketosis: getting it accustomed to burning fat instead of glucose. You'll lose more weight on your round of HCG if your body gets this running start on ketosis.

This process is called becoming "fat adapted." It's a quick start to the longer-term ketogenic diet, which uses a low carbohydrate / high healthy fat diet to keep you in ketosis. For now, think of the loading phase as flipping the switch that puts your body into ketosis. The HCG Loading Phase prepares your body to burn fat more effectively throughout the diet.

The basic guideline for the Loading Phase is that your calories and fat will be *high* but your starches and sugars (carbohydrates) will be *low*. Keeping your carbs very low, despite eating a lot of food, is called "loading clean."

Loading Clean

When you're in the loading phase, it's tempting to eat all the foods you know you will miss over the next few months. You will be able to eat a lot of delicious food these two days, but *during the loading phase, your best bet is to focus on rich, fatty foods that are low carb.*

Try brie cheese, bacon, pulled pork, short ribs, veggies cooked in butter or oil, salmon, macadamia nuts, bratwurst, avocado with blue cheese dressing, asparagus and poached eggs with hollandaise sauce, whipping cream or coconut milk in your coffee (and so on).

You can eat fried foods, but not if they're breaded or battered in the traditional way. You could fry chicken tenders or fish sticks in a coating of crushed pork rinds and parmesan cheese, for example (super delicious and crispy) but not in a coating of bread crumbs, cracker crumbs or panko.

Avoid vegetable oils like canola, safflower, sunflower, grape seed, palm seed and corn oil. All of these make it more difficult to lose weight, because their Omega 6 fatty acids cause inflammation. Choose instead to fry in fats that are not inflammatory: avocado oil, coconut oil, olive oil, peanut oil, almond oil, ghee, pork lard, beef tallow, chicken schmaltz, butter and duck fat. Some people would quibble with peanut oil being on this list for your long term health, as it's not as anti-inflammatory as animal fats are, for example. However peanut oil is good enough — it's readily available, has a high smoke point and tastes delicious; it's fine for the loading phase.

Adding fat is the fun part of the loading phase. The hard part is avoiding foods that are mostly starch or sugar. Avoid anything made with grains or legumes, like rice, beans, oats, wheat, spelt and corn, as well as high-carb seeds such as quinoa. Obviously, avoid baked goods made with any of these flours, including gluten-free items. Your best bet is to steer clear of processed foods for these few days. Other foods to avoid on the loading phase are winter squash, potatoes and other root vegetables, most fresh fruit and all dried fruit.

A good approach to the loading phase is to think in advance of foods that are high fat and low starch. Unsweetened chocolate is one of those foods. So is cream cheese. So is guacamole. So are chicken wings made without breading. The **salt & vinegar wings at**

Buffalo Wild Wings work, as do garlic-parmesan wings you bake at home using pork rinds and grated cheese as your crisp crust.

During the loading phase, the goal is not to eat as many calories as you can; it's to eat as large a percentage of fat as you can. Your healthcare provider should help you set a caloric goal for your loading phase. For women, the goal is likely to be around 2,200 - 2,300 calories.

The original Simeons protocol stresses the importance of patients "gorging" during the loading phase, even to the point of nausea. But the thing is, 2,300 calories isn't all that much if you're eating ribs, brie and avocado and putting heavy cream in your coffee. Don't think of the loading phase as a time to go wild, think of it as a time to be strategic about getting into ketosis.

Needless to say, we don't believe it's essential for you to feel nauseous. We assume that Dr. Simeons meant that patients often feel nauseous when they have eaten a fattier diet than usual — that is very true. If you do feel nauseous, it probably means you did a good job of overwhelming your digestive system with your fat intake for the day. Neither gorging nor nausea are vital to succeeding on the HCG loading phase, though. In fact, you'll probably feel more motivated for the low calorie phase if you aren't feeling gross.

Dr. Simeons also discouraged patients from skipping the loading phase. He observed that some patients try to skip the initial weight gain, thinking it's a clever strategy for maximum weight loss. He was right: that's not a good strategy. Don't skip the loading phase, because it's vital to your body losing the most stored fat possible. We hope you agree it's worth the anxiety of gaining a few pounds in order to lose many more pounds.

Examples of food decision-making during the loading phase:

Triple creme brie? **Yes.**

     On crackers? **No.**

Baby back ribs? **Yes.**

     With sweet BBQ sauce? **No.**

Whipping cream in your coffee? **Yes.**

     Plus caramel syrup? **No.**

Omelette with extra yolk and cheese? **Yes.**

     Side of hash browns? **No.**

Granola of coconut, macadamias, pecans and pork rinds? **Yes.**

     Add dried apricots, oats and honey? **No.**

Poached eggs with ham and hollandaise? **Yes.**

     On an English muffin? **No.**

Chorizo, pork carnitas or beef barbacoa? **Yes.**

     In a tortilla? **No.**

Consider choosing the parts of your favorite dishes that will work for the loading phase (let's say a bacon cheeseburger) and leaving out the ingredients that would work against you due to high starch or sugar (ketchup, brioche bun). To make your own HCG ketchup, honey mustard or sweet pickle relish without sugar, read the section "Tricks with Alternative Natural Sweeteners."

Metabolic Complexity and Sense of Humor

When you're on HCG, keeping your sense of humor will be a huge asset. Your resilience will be useful because eating so carefully can feel little crazy, but also because our endocrine system is so complicated. Here are some things to bear in mind about metabolic function when trying to lose weight.

Maintain your eye for the absurd

Counting calories, calculating protein ratios and weighing portions is intense and a little nutty. It would be easy to get perfectionistic and lose the big picture; please don't do that. If you made healthy **mu-shu chicken with cabbage, mushrooms, bamboo shoots and chicken breast** but ate too much of it, that doesn't undo all of your hard work. If you took a few bites of the cranberry scone your colleague baked, accidentally ate ketchup made with corn syrup or went over your calories for the day, it doesn't undo all of your hard work. Overall, you're still doing great. Don't let fluctuations break your stride.

You attended a Cinco de Mayo party and brought chicken tikka masala and iced cardamom tea from home because you can't have guacamole, pork adobo tacos or margaritas right now. It's remarkable what you did for yourself! It's also a little bit funny that you're eating Indian food at a Cinco de Mayo party. Keep that eye for the absurd. You were willing to bring your own chicken breast, even though you would have liked a pork taco.

Especially when you're on HCG, your body would know the difference between those two dishes in their fat content. Your efforts matter.

Is a pickle a meal?

Under normal circumstances, a single pickle would not be a compelling meal. We're accustomed to eating a main event, like a sandwich, maybe a fun side dish like fries, maybe a virtuous side dish like a green salad, then perhaps a soda and something sweet at the end. When you're on HCG, you will be happiest if you think more broadly about what constitutes a meal. It's a simple attitude adjustment that may prevent you from being too literal about your eating.

For example, if you're at a deli, and you need something that's not fatty meat like pastrami or a mayonnaise-based side dish like potato salad, look for the humongous barrel of **Kosher dill pickles**. On that particular day — for you — a pickle is a meal.

That example is a helpful metaphor for the HCG Diet. You'll probably have a few experiences like this, when you reach dinner time with very few calories remaining. Prioritize finding something that manages your hunger, rather than something that's a suitable "dinner." You may find that on some days, you eat swordfish for breakfast, radishes for lunch and egg whites for dinner. Allow your meals to be weird while on Phase 2.

Yogurt is not the devil

One of the reasons it's so vital to keep things in perspective while on HCG is that what's happening metabolically is hugely complex. *When the scale plateaus or goes up, it doesn't mean that you're not losing fat.* For example, some people see the scale jump because they have a food sensitivity they weren't aware of.

Let's say someone is sensitive to cow dairy, even though they're not technically "lactose intolerant." If they don't have symptoms that are obvious to them and have never been tested for food sensitivities, they probably wouldn't know that their body doesn't appreciate cow dairy. (Since some of our food intolerances don't develop until adulthood, this example is a common one.) If that person eats a little Greek yogurt or cottage cheese while on HCG, it could cause them to retain water, bringing them up a pound or two the next day.

If that person didn't realize it was just the *dairy* they ate, causing an inflammatory response, they might think it was real weight they had gained. The Greek yogurt may have been the culprit, but that doesn't mean you can never eat it again; it just means that fresh cow dairy is a risky choice for you at the moment. Don't let it get you down.

Constant exposure to food sensitivities makes the lining of the small intestines more permeable, allowing food across this barrier. Believe it or not, 70% of our immune system resides beneath the lining of the gut. So you can imagine that when the gut is exposed to challenging foods, there are problems downstream, so to speak. The "weight gain" we see when people eat foods they are sensitive to is actually systemic inflammation — a signal that the immune system, within that gut lining, has been compromised.

If you decide that monitoring your food sensitivities on top of everything else you're tracking is just too much, that's fine. What you're doing is already an impressive amount of work. If you do decide to investigate your food sensitivities, there's a how-to section later in this book, called "Guide to Testing Food Sensitivities."

How often you eat matters

Did you know that how *often* you eat matters, too? This is quite contemporary research about the effects of insulin, so we wouldn't expect someone seeing patients in 1954, like Dr. Simeons was, to have been aware of this dimension.

Dr. Simeons recommended skipping breakfast or having just coffee/tea in the morning. In Italy, it is common to have just an espresso drink for breakfast; there's a cultural basis for his recommendation. We now know, though, that our insulin sensitivity is at its *best* in the morning and its worst in the evening. In other words, if you were to skip a meal when trying to lose weight, dinner would be your wisest choice, not breakfast.

The bottom line is that you needn't have just coffee or tea for breakfast while on P2, unless you want to. We're not encouraging you to skip dinner, we're just saying that metabolically, it's not necessary to limit breakfast to zero-calorie beverages while on Phase 2.

Interestingly, how many times per day you eat affects how easily you lose weight, too. Eating fewer times is better, because your body has an insulin response each time you give it food. Research has shown that subjects who ate two meals a day, with no snacking between, lost more adiposity (fat) and maintained more muscle mass than subjects who consumed *the same number of calories* but ate throughout the day (Martinez-Lopez, et.al, 2017). Interesting, huh? It's easier to lose weight if you contain eating to as few "events" as possible, rather than grazing throughout the day.

That said, you'll have so few calories to work with during P2, you may need to snack to manage hunger; that's okay. For now, it's not essential that you eat in as few sittings as possible. If you're interested in the absolute most effective way to burn fat, though, eating fewer times per day is the ideal.

How long you eat matters

Some people choose to eat an early dinner, with no snacking afterwards, then a late breakfast. Leaving a prolonged time between these two meals essentially creates a fasting period. When people compress the number of hours per day they eat, it's called Time-Restricted Eating (TRE). For example, if you ate only between the hours of 10:00am and 6:00pm, we'd say your "eating window" for that day was eight hours. Limiting the number of hours we eat per day is much better for weight loss than having a very long eating window is.

Time-Restricted Eating is helpful because it gives your liver and pancreas a break from processing insulin. During the hours you aren't eating, they have some down time. This down time enables your liver to devote more energy to fat burning (Panda, 2018.)

The research is ongoing, but it appears that the benefits of time-restricted eating kick in at about 12 hours without food; much more so at 14 hours. If someone finished dinner at 7:00pm, and had nothing more that evening (other than tea, coffee, still or sparkling water, salt, medications) at 7:00am the next morning it would be a 12 hour fast. At 9:00am it would be a 14 hour fast. That's not what most people think of as "fasting," but to your endocrine system it's very helpful. This is especially true if you want to lose weight. People who are keen to do Time Restricted Eating usually aim to allow 14 or more hours between dinner and breakfast.

Another benefit of time-restricted eating is that it gives the body an opportunity to clean waste and recycle proteins; a physiological renewal of sorts called autophagy. Some people drive autophagy most effectively with mild or moderate exercise in the fasting state, but this is likely something you'd not explore until after the HCG Diet. You should first be cleared by a healthcare professional if you want to exercise while on a very low calorie diet.

Time-Restricted Eating is not necessary when you are on HCG; it's tough enough to eat so few calories without worrying about what time you finished dinner! But FYI, if you choose to keep your eating window more narrow than the entire day, it will maximize your results.

Metabolism beyond calories

Vital to keeping your sense of humor is remembering that there are many, many factors at play with weight fluctuations. This is true of our everyday metabolic function and is especially true when taking an exogenous hormone, like human chorionic gonadotropin.

Our endocrine system is paying attention to all sorts of information, not just how many calories we consumed and how many we burned off. To repeat: our weight is not just about the number of calories we took in versus the number of calories we expended. This is entirely different from what we learned in middle school health class, isn't it? Body weight is hormonal; there's plenty of empirical evidence for this. Don't be terribly concerned if you go over your caloric goal for the day.

We encourage you to maintain a rigorous curiosity about how complex metabolic processes are, rather than getting spooked by the arithmetic of calories. Be rigorous in your eye for the absurd. Yesterday you ate 603 calories and today your weight is up 1/2 pound? That is nuts! But it's not, actually; that's the point here. Your body is responding to far more variables than what you ate on a single day.

What we discuss next is vital to your mental preparation for HCG. It's about how people who have been overweight a long time burn fat differently from those who've not been overweight for very long.

Individual Differences in Fat Metabolism

We used to think that if we consume fewer calories than we expend, we will lose weight; end of story. It turns out that's such a vast over-simplification, it's essentially incorrect.

Did you know that just a modest number of carbs can set off fluid retention, inflammation and weight gain in some people? That information never appeared on the food pyramid with the drawings of wheat and corn, did it? The body's over-reaction to half a peach or a little hummus doesn't happen to everyone, only to people who are very carb-sensitive, like those with diabetes and pre-diabetes. It can also affect people who have been overweight for many years.

If there are factors other than calories and exercise in the mix, what are those things? What accounts for individual differences in the way we metabolize fat? One of the most potent factors is how healthy a person's fat cells are.

The nature of fat

The root of clinical obesity is this: not all fat cells are alike. The type of fat cells that grow in obese mammals, including humans, are atypical. The current term in medicine for this condition is adiposopathy or "sick fat disease." Sick fat cells act more like glandular tissue than they do like fat cells. They are supposed to simply *store* excess calories, but sick fat cells actually *produce* hormones and inflammation that encourage fat production.

To repeat: people with clinical obesity produce fat more easily than healthy patients do, because their fat cells work differently. People who are healthy metabolically are less prone to storing fat, regardless of what they eat. In fact, overweight people often eat less than slender people do! You probably knew that intuitively. The conventional "calories in/calories out" model of weight loss is especially incorrect for people with clinical obesity.

Fat cells do not have calorie receptors. They respond to what we eat, when we eat and how much we eat, but it's not the same formula for every person. All calories aren't the same once they're on the inside. That makes sense when you think about it — 300 calories of potato is processed quite differently from 300 calories of salmon. Not only that, we each inherit a unique set of metabolic strengths and weaknesses from our parents. It's much more complicated than calories minus exercise = pant size.

Public health data point to the early 1980s as the start of our obesity epidemic in the United States. This coincides with the introduction of reduced-fat and sugar-free products. Many of these products are higher in carbohydrate than is healthy, but for years we were told that saturated fat was the heart of the problem. We followed that bouncing ball to reduced fat cookies, rice cakes and fat free sour cream. Yikes. Saturated fat, which causes very little insulin response, is not what causes obesity. Fat + carbohydrate will make you gain weight, but fat alone? No. That's the premise of ketogenic science.

Fortunately, obesity is now a recognized disease state. A person's size should never trigger judgment of their character or effort. Unfortunately, many people who live with clinical obesity still don't know that it's a metabolic disease and do judge themselves.

Leptin resistance

Another example of individual differences in fat metabolism is leptin resistance. If you don't feel full at the end of a good-sized meal or if you find yourself grazing after dinner but not feeling especially hungry early in the day, you may have leptin resistance.

The hormone leptin is typically secreted by the gut after a meal. It is supposed to tickle the hypothalamus, signaling that the stomach is full, which triggers a feeling of fullness.

People with excess visceral fat sometimes produce too much leptin. When this happens, the leptin in their blood may be high even when they're fasting. The hypothalamus is receiving fullness messages constantly. Because satiety signals are being sent too often, they are eventually ignored by the brain. Thus we become *resistant* to leptin. After a while, that person cannot feel when they are actually physiologically hungry and when they are not.

To repeat: some people eat more than they need to because their brain doesn't get the message that they are satisfied — and this metabolic condition is more common among people with excess visceral fat. Leptin resistance is pretty torturous when you're trying to lose weight, because you constantly feel hungry.

Reducing visceral fat heals leptin resistance. The very low calorie phase of the HCG Diet (Phase 2) can help reset the brain's ability to register accurate signals that you are full.

Fat cells and toxins

Environmental toxins can make our fat cells sick, too. New chemicals are constantly introduced in clothing, air, pre-packaged foods (even some organic foods), lotions, hair products, cosmetics and beverages. Those sick fat cells then become *mutagenic fat*; they have mutated in response to environmental toxins.

There's an entire class of chemicals toxicologists call "obesogens." These are chemicals that once stored in our cells (mostly in fat cells) force them to perform differently. Instead of these fat cells providing storage, as they should, they begin to produce inflammatory mediators and hormones! This includes leptin, which confuses our hunger signals, and estrogen, which is associated with weight gain. Why blather on about environmental toxins? Because it helps explain why obesity is a disease, not a weakness.

The more atypical fat cells a person has, the more sensitive they become to sweetness and starch. Of course, people with years of clinical obesity have more of these mutated cells. Again: people who are overweight have fat cells that overreact to sweetness and starch. Their body reacts to carbohydrate by causing cravings, so you'll feed it more of that substance. That's a different reaction to food than someone whose fat cells are healthy.

It's a vicious cycle. You know how the rich get richer and the poor get poorer? The same principle applies to metabolism: the fat get fatter, because their cells respond differently to the food they eat. The more fat you have, the more vulnerable you are to accumulating more of it. It's so unfair. This is why we strongly suggest you make your P2 food choices with carbohydrate grams in mind, not just calorie count or a set list.

Constipation

We've discussed the negative effects of environmental toxins on fat cells, but you can detox in a way that's deeply satisfying: try to have a well-formed bowel movement every day. Constipation is pretty common on the HCG Diet. Here are some strategies that may help you to "detoxify."

1. Take 25 grams of fiber daily. This can come from food and/or from the fiber supplements we discuss in the section "Tips for Pushing Through Hunger," such as **PGX fiber**.

2. Hydrate well. Shoot for drinking one-half of your body weight in ounces of water + an additional cup for any caffeinated beverage you drink (they are diuretics).

3. Increase the amount of walking you do.

4. Mix **magnesium citrate powder** into your water. Use 200-1000mg per day. Begin at a low dose.

5. Buy some *Smooth Move Tea* by Traditional Medicinals or *Get Regular Tea* by Yogi. Both have a little senna in them, which in small amounts is a gentle remedy for constipation. Smooth Move's original version tastes like licorice, and both brands come in a mint flavor, as well.

Limit your use of anything with a laxative effect to several times per week, as there's some risk of dependence on it. Ethical dilemma: Serve as iced tea to someone who's not supporting you?

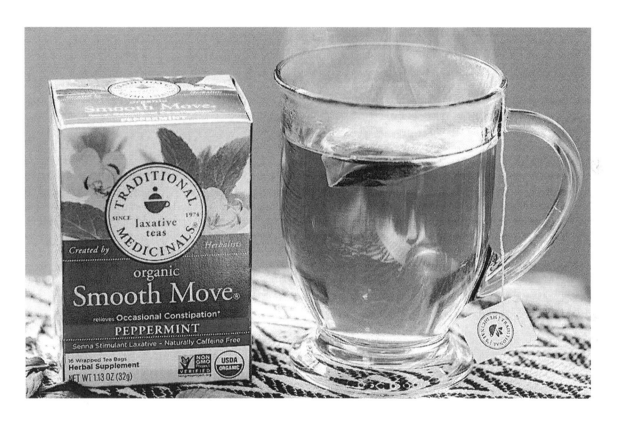

Low carbohydrate diets can be constipating, as can low fat diets. HCG is both of these things, for a short time! Take it as a sign of success if you get a little backed up. Constipation makes the scale move more slowly, so don't fret.

6. Take a sauna, if that's an option. Sweating is a great way to eliminate toxins, but if you do, be sure to add a **high quality electrolyte powder** to water to replenish nutrients. You'll know that you're overdue for electrolytes if you feel light-headed, dizzy or have muscle cramps.

Metabolism changes with age

Men and women both find it more difficult to lose weight as they age. Some people are genetically predisposed to a better metabolism, though, even into mid-life, which gives them some wiggle room with their diet as they age. Other people have metabolic disorders, such as diabetes, which makes it more difficult for them to lose weight in general, but especially as they age. Of course menopause poses a special challenge for women trying to achieve a healthy body weight.

In her excellent book *The Wisdom of Menopause* (2012) Dr. Christiane Northrup describes how menopause affects metabolism and weight loss. Beginning with perimenopause, when a woman's period has become irregular, metabolism is affected because estrogen is affected.

During menopause, the balance between estrogen and progesterone may be thrown off. If estrogen is not moderated by progesterone, the result is called estrogen dominance. When this happens, a chain reaction may lead to low thyroid hormones.

When a person has inadequate thyroid hormones, their metabolism typically goes down. This is a simplified picture of hypothyroid (that's fully explained in Dr. Northrup's book) but the bottom line is that you may want to have your thyroid function examined.

If you are near menopause or past it and have noticed you gain weight even while trying to lose it, consider discussing this with your physician. If (s)he believes it's warranted, a metabolic panel may be ordered. This blood work would include tests of your thyroid function. It may be that medications or supplements could help balance your hormones.

Interestingly, Dr. Northrup also makes mention of ketosis as a way to break through weight loss stalls at menopause. She notes that a very low carbohydrate diet, such as the Atkins Diet, is useful. This reinforces the notion that HCG, and later a ketogenic diet, addresses fat metabolism.

For now, just bear in mind that there are individual differences in the way people process fat. How healthy your fat cells are, how sensitive you are to leptin and how your hormones respond to the life cycle will vary among us. It's not a straightforward process.

Alternative natural sweeteners

A brief overview of alternative natural sweeteners:

1. They're better than sugar and artificial sweeteners are
2. In small doses, they're safe for most on HCG
3. They come in various solid and liquid forms
4. They vary in terms of how sweet they are
5. People vary by how well their tummy tolerates them

Our bodies respond quite differently to *natural sugars* (like honey, agave, maple syrup and cane sugar) than they do to *artificial sweeteners* (like aspartame, sucralose, saccharin and maltitol) and *alternative natural sweeteners* (like stevia, erythritol, monk fruit, allulose and xylitol).

Natural sugars and artificial sweeteners may cause spikes of insulin and blood glucose, so they work against weight loss. (In fact, some would say that aspartame in a diet soda is no better for you than sugar or corn syrup is in a regular soda!) If you choose to use sweeteners while on HCG, *alternative natural sweeteners* are your safest bet.

Some people stay away from all sweeteners, even alternative natural sweeteners, while on HCG and that's a fine choice. If that is what you do, remember that there are a few delicious fruits that are low enough in carbohydrate to be safe for HCG. Casaba melon (Tier 2) and watermelon (Tier 3) are sweet and juicy. Dice them small, freeze them, then crush the frozen fruit in your food processor or blender. Add a little water or iced tea to make a damn good **melon sorbet.** Add a larger amount of liquid to make a **melon slushy drink**.

Even "natural sugars" are sugar

Obviously you would not eat granulated sugar while on HCG, but what about other natural sugars?

All of the following ingredients are natural substances that metabolically are sugar:

Agave, balsamic vinegar, brown rice syrup, carob syrup, coconut sugar, corn syrup, date syrup, evaporated cane juice, fresh or dried fruit, fruit juice, golden syrup, honey, maple sugar, maple syrup, molasses, palm sugar, pure cane juice, raw turbinado sugar, treacle.

Avoid all of these sugars while on HCG. They can kick you out of ketosis.

Read labels for hidden sugars

No newsflash here: sweetness makes food taste good. Even foods that are spicy, sour, salty savory or umami generally taste better with some sweetness in the mix. Since consumers read labels more often than they used to, manufacturers have gotten pretty good at listing ingredients we will not recognize as sugars. This practice especially holds true for fat-free products, which may have higher than average sugars to compensate for the flavor and texture the fat provided.

You don't want hidden sugars if you're trying to lose weight, especially when on HCG.

Keep an eye out for these ingredients on food labels:

Barbados sugar, barley malt, beet sugar, buttered syrup, cane juice, caramel, carob syrup, castor sugar, corn syrup, date sugar, dehydrated cane juice, dextran, dextrose, diabetic malt, diastase, ethyl malt, fructose, fruit juice, fruit juice concentrate, glucose solids, grape sugar, high fructose corn syrup, invert sugar, lactose, malt, malt syrup, maltitol, maltodextrin, maltose, molasses, muscovado, panocha, refiner's syrup, rice syrup, sorbitol, sorghum syrup and sucrose.

Artificial sweeteners are risky, too

Artificial sweeteners have been in our lives for decades. Examples of these sweeteners are aspartame, saccharin, sorbitol, sucralose and maltitol. Brand names include Sweet n' Low (saccharin), Splenda (sucralose) and Equal (aspartame). Artificial sweeteners seemed so promising at first. Tab instead of Coke!

In recent years, we've come to understand that like sugar, artificial sweeteners may cause a blood sugar spike and/or an insulin response. Both of these processes work against weight loss. Artificial sweeteners also tend to increase hunger and some have a laxative effect. Sorbitol and maltitol are notorious for causing stomach upset.

There are more serious issues than keeping you close to the restroom. Sucralose for example may disturb thyroid function and block iodine absorption. Sucralose is not a naturally occurring compound, so it's a molecule the human body is unfamiliar with. That molecule is hundreds of times sweeter than sugar. Sucralose binds to our taste buds and remains longer than sugar does, so it has a more profound effect on metabolism and cravings than sugar does.

In short, steer clear of products made with sucralose or Splenda while on HCG. You'd be better off eating some fruit, despite its carbs, than you would be using any sweetener that threatens to mess with your metabolism and cravings.

Alternative natural sweeteners in small amounts

The opportunity to add a *little* sweetness can expand your cooking repertoire quite a bit. Unlike artificial sweeteners, which are chemically engineered, alternative natural sweeteners are plant-based. Read the section below, "Alternative Natural Sweeteners to Consider" for examples of your options.

Alternative natural sweeteners generally do not cause a spike in your blood sugar, but they may still cause an insulin response. This means they're not "freebies" metabolically, but they are a safer choice for you than sugar and artificial sweeteners are. Our approach is that a little bit of alternative natural sweetener is okay on HCG if you use it to prevent yourself from going off-plan.

Here's the bummer: for people who have metabolic issues, even alternative natural sweeteners may pose a threat to weight loss. Whether or not you've been formally diagnosed with Type II Diabetes, it's possible you have had glucose intolerance, insulin resistance, leptin resistance or other conditions. Alternative natural sweeteners are more likely to spike hormones for patients with these issues, slowing their weight loss.

If you're on the very low calorie phase of the diet and are relying pretty heavily upon alternative natural sweeteners, conduct a science experiment: eat the same number of calories as usual, but remove sweeteners for two days. Does this increase the rate of your weight loss or get you unstuck from a stall? If it does, that's awfully useful data! Though we can't be certain the weight change is due to eliminating sweeteners (since you probably didn't eat precisely the same food every day) chances are good that's the answer; it's the answer for many patients.

If you suspect you'd get better weight loss results by removing alternative natural sweeteners, but know that having no sweetness is not realistic for you, a nice substitute would be some low glycemic fruit, like **strawberries, raspberries or blackberries**.

You might also limit your sweeteners to a couple of drops of **stevia glycerite** in your hot coffee or chai tea with MCT oil each day.

Refer to the section called "Flavor Tricks with Alternative Natural Sweeteners" to inspire some cooking ideas. Making homemade ketchup, for example, is a huge help.

Diet sodas made with alternative natural sweeteners

Although sweeteners of any kind are not ideal for maximizing weight loss, a good diet soda can really hit the spot when on P2; they do serve a purpose.

If you'd like a diet soda while on HCG, try **Zevia sodas** (sweetened with stevia) or **Dry Soda Zero Sugar** (sweetened with erythritol) rather than the usual diet beverages sweetened with aspartame, sucralose or another artificial sweetener. Zevia and Dry Soda Zero Sugar are available in some upscale supermarkets, but you will have the widest choice of their flavors by purchasing online. Personal favorites: Dry Soda Mountain Berry and Ruby Citrus flavors. Zevia cola and tonic water flavors.

Alternative Natural Sweeteners to Consider

Alternative natural sweeteners vary in terms of how sweet they are; some are far sweeter than sugar is, making them tricky to cook with. Sweeteners also vary in form: you'll find liquid drops, syrups, granular, powdered and "brown sugar" forms. Alternative natural sweeteners also vary in terms of how gut-friendly they are — more on this below.

Here is a rundown of some alternative natural sweeteners on the market at the time of this writing. It's common for products to be blends of several sweeteners.

Swerve is a very good choice. It's erythritol + oligosaccharide. It comes in granulated, powdered and "brown sugar" forms, tastes good and measures 1:1 like sugar. Tummy problems are rare with Swerve. Some markets actually carry Swerve on their shelves.

Sukrin is erythritol + stevia. This product comes in granulated, powdered and "brown sugar" forms; it has no aftertaste and measures 1:1 like sugar. Sukrin Classic is like white sugar and Sukrin Melis is like powdered sugar. Sukrin fiber syrup is an excellent product — it's thick like honey or corn syrup but not overly sweet. Sukrin is typically ordered online.

All-u-lose and *Wholesome* are brands of allulose sold in plain liquid and granular forms. Allulose is less sweet than sugar and it caramelizes, which offers a special advantage for browning foods.

All-u-lose Brand makes a maple-flavored syrup and a honey-flavored syrup that are remarkably good. For HCG purposes, either of these would make for a mighty fine "honey mustard" if mixed with plain mustard. Allulose is what's called a rare sugar and some tummies don't tolerate it well, but for those that do, it's a gem.

Stevia glycerite or *"Better Stevia"* by Now Foods is a versatile player. It's a thicker, less concentrated form of stevia drops so it's easier to control in recipes. Stevia glycerite has less aftertaste than regular stevia drops do and has no bitterness, the way some powdered forms of stevia do. Many people also like ***Sweet Leaf* stevia drops** when on P2, because they come in flavors like berry, orange, lemon, apricot, chocolate and vanilla creme.

Lakanto is monk fruit extract + erythritol. It comes in drops, granular white, granular golden, powdered and maple syrup forms. Lakanto's drops and powdered version are quite sweet; the granular forms are easier to work with. Lakanto granular is more coarse in texture than some brands are, so it has crunch. We've heard people say that they appreciate Golden Lakanto in particular, because it has some caramel notes. You might **pulverize Golden Lakanto in your coffee bean grinder** to create a powdered sweetener that's not overly sweet and has those caramel notes. This way you can really disperse the flavor without using much of it.

Like Lakanto, ***Choc Zero*** uses monk fruit extract to sweeten. Consumers typically rate Choc Zero products extremely high for authentic flavor without aftertaste. You won't be able to explore their chocolate chips, chocolate bark or peanut butter cups while on HCG, but you could use any of their **sugar free syrups in flavors like caramel, coconut, peach, maple, maple-pecan and chocolate.**

Plain erythritol is granular and is inexpensive, as is **plain Xylitol**. Both are versatile alternative natural sweeteners. A few considerations, though: plain erythritol leaves a slightly cooling taste in the mouth. Xylitol is highly toxic to house pets. Overall though, both of these sweeteners are useful, economical choices.

If you decide to use some alternative natural sweeteners, you'll find them easily online. Websites such as vitacost.com, netrition.com, thrivemarket.com and amazon.com are all good resources.

Use in Case of Emergency

If alternative natural sweeteners like erythritol are safe for P2, why do we have to be cautious about the amount we use? They're risky because their sweetness stimulates the brain in much the same way sugar does — they may increase hunger and cause sugar cravings.

Alternative natural sweeteners cause your pancreas to release insulin. Insulin instructs your body to *store* fat. The HCG hormone instructs your body to *burn* stored fat. You'd be giving your body conflicting messages.

Finally, sweeteners may cause bloating, inflammation and water retention. If this happens, it will temporarily stall your weight loss. That's so discouraging when you're doing everything else right!

Taken together, we suggest using alternative natural sweeteners "in case of emergency." Leaning heavily on them is not a good strategy, but some patients say that using them sparingly in their cooking enables them to stick with Phase 2. A touch of sweetener to make a salad dressing or a gelatin dessert, for example, may help with sticking to the diet.

Finding the right sweetener

Some people tolerate stevia drops well, with no gastrointestinal upset, but they don't like the slight bitter aftertaste. Some people like allulose, which tastes great and caramelizes well, but it makes them nauseous. Some people appreciate that erythritol doesn't upset their tummy but they dislike that it has a slight cooling sensation. Some people like the flavor of monk fruit sweeteners best, but it makes them fart like a bulldog, so they select something else. As with so many things in life, it's a trade-off.

You may need to purchase several brands of alternative natural sweetener and give them a trial run. Making this a part of your preparation process for the HCG Diet would be time and money well-spent. If you'd like to try just one sweetener and play it by ear, you might begin with **Swerve Confectioners**.

Fat-free products

Fat free products are generally higher in carbs than their normal equivalents are. Fat-free yogurt, for example, usually has more carbohydrate than whole milk yogurt does. While it's true you'll want foods that are low in fat while on P2, you'll want foods that are *naturally* low in fat, not engineered to be that way.

In a pinch, you can have a few tablespoonfuls of **nonfat yogurt** on HCG, especially if it's the difference between sticking to the low calorie phase and giving up. For example, if you add dehydrated onion flakes, a little pickle brine and some fresh dill to non-fat plain yogurt, you've got a **dip for raw veggies or a "mayo"** to make leftover turkey salad less dry.

Gluten free products

The ingredients used in gluten-free products are sometimes higher in carbohydrate than the traditional versions of those foods are. Don't go looking for gluten-free Melba toast; it's *grain*-free products you need.

To illustrate: rice flour is gluten free. So are chickpea flour, oat flour, amaranth flour, millet flour and lentil flour. These all work beautifully for gluten-free baking and breading, so they are a terrific help for people with Celiac Disease, but they're not useful for ketosis. Gluten-free flours have just as much carbohydrate as glutinous flours like wheat, rye, spelt, barley and kamut do. For weight loss purposes, being *grain*-free is what's important, not being gluten-free.

Some products are both gluten free *and* grain free, which sounds promising, but the problem is that tapioca starch and potato starch are often used as binders. These are still high in carbohydrate, so not good for HCG. The same is true for ground seeds and legumes, like quinoa flour and lentil flour, which are grain free and gluten free, but not low in carbohydrate. Your concern during P2 should be the carbohydrate and fat content of your food choices, not whether they have gluten.

A good workaround for pasta is spaghetti squash, which is a Tier 2 veggie. Spaghetti squash doesn't have much flavor (which is a virtue in this case) and it really does look like spaghetti. Try **spaghetti squash baked with cinnamon and allspice** as a side dish.

MCT Oil

MCT oil is a highly strained form of coconut oil. Remarkably, medium chain triglycerides (MCTs) help your body access stored fat and use it for fuel. Since accessing our stored body fat is the entire point of taking the HCG hormone, they work beautifully together.

It may seem illogical to add oil to a period of low oil consumption. Here are some frequently asked questions about MCT oil:

Yes, you may have MCT oil in Phase 2, in liquid or powder form.
No, you can't consume regular coconut oil.

Yes, there's a recommended amount: 2 tbs MCT oil per day.
No, you don't need to count these calories!

Yes, you may create pesto, vinaigrettes and creamy hot beverages.
No, you can't use MCT oil to sauté or fry. It has a very low smoke point.

Yes, you may have a little bit more than 2 tbs per day, if you wish. Up to 3 tbs.
No, you can't have an unlimited amount of MCT oil. You'd poop like a goose.

Yes, the best way to avoid stomach upset is to work gradually up to 3 tbs.

Good MCT oil is an expensive supplement, but patients who use it typically lose more weight than those who don't. Adding a few tablespoons of MCT oil spikes your serum fat level. This up-regulates the enzymes that break down body fat for fuel. In other words, MCT oil facilitates ketosis and increases metabolism — both of which are precisely what we want.

MCT oil often causes diarrhea in the beginning, so work your way up to the full dose. As described in the "Twenty Preparations for HCG" chapter, you might begin building your tolerance for MCT oil even before Phase 2 of the diet.

Since you can only consume 2-3 tablespoons MCT oil per day without spending the evening in misery, you'll need to think about what recipe you'd like to "spend" your daily MCT oil on. Some people use it for a **"honey mustard" vinaigrette** to make a cole slaw, tuna salad or turkey salad. Others like to use it in hot beverages to make them creamy, like a **chai tea or a latte**. Some make a room temperature **pesto they use to dress hot vegetables**, like a watercress pesto (which is naturally spicy).

The highest heat MCT oil can tolerate is about 320° F (Emmerich & Emmerich, 2018) so it's fine for adding to your warm beverage, making a **warm dressing for a spinach salad or a warm pesto for your broccoli.** Usually we bake and stir-fry at temperatures above 320 degrees, so MCT oil is not often used in these applications. You could certainly experiment with sautéing dishes at medium-low to see what you can create, though. A piece of white fish that dries out easily, like halibut, would probably work fine in a 315 degree oven, topped with your homemade **lemon-garlic MCT pesto.**

After HCG, you might actually be eating a diet that's *rich* in healthy fats. If you choose to transition to the ketogenic diet, you may use MCT oil for maintaining ketosis. See the section "Continuing a Ketogenic Lifestyle" if interested in this jumpstart. For the present though, the only fat that will work in your favor on Phase 2 is MCT oil.

Alcohol

You're no dummy. You know that alcohol doesn't work for P2. Your liver will be working exceptionally hard on your behalf to address fat metabolism and detoxifying. Since the liver addresses alcohol before it addresses fat, drinking will slow fat burning. Giving your liver more to contend with always works against weight loss, not just while on HCG.

That said, can you have a sip of wine at a special dinner or taste the craft beer your friend has made without it becoming a runaway train? Some people who aren't in recovery are able to do so. If that's you, a sip of alcohol will not undo all of your work, but it may slow your progress. Think of it this way: drinking alcohol on HCG is like eating cotton candy when the goal is to lower your blood sugar.

We're fairly sure that alcohol also has a negative impact on glycemic control and insulin action. That's how much your liver produces the hormone that directs fat storage. Steiner, Crowell & Lang (2015) point this out, though they also acknowledge that the research is not yet conclusive.

Of course, alcohol is also calorie-dense and not filling, so it doesn't make much sense while on the HCG hormone. If you do drink, bear in mind that when eating low carb, it may take less alcohol for you to become intoxicated. If you choose to consume alcohol while on HCG, choose drinks that cause a relatively low insulin response: pure spirits like gin, vodka and whiskey and dry wines or brut champagne all have a lower glycemic index than beer, hard cider, wine coolers, liqueurs and cocktails made with mixers do.

Tips for Pushing Through Hunger

Managing hunger is something you could actually rehearse before your round of HCG. That may sound goofy, but once you begin the very low calorie phase, already knowing what works for you may be helpful.

What decreases your hunger pangs just enough for you to fall asleep? What would help when you've just eaten a tiny meal and are still hungry? Which of the strategies suggested here work for other people but not for you? Might you devise some strategy that becomes a reliable go-to? Perhaps a **hibiscus tea slushy** or a **pineapple seltzer with coconut stevia drops** really hits the spot for you. In general, unsweetened seltzer that's coconut, pineapple or coconut-pineapple tastes great with a drops of stevia that are vanilla or coconut flavored. The result **tastes like cream soda**.

Below are some experiments for pushing through hunger, but talk with your healthcare provider if the intensity of your hunger is more than 6 out of 10 while on HCG; the hormone is supposed to manage appetite fairly well. There's a relatively narrow window of effective dosing on HCG, so yours may be too high or too low if you feel like you're starving.

Beverages

Seltzer water is filling and comes in many subtle, unsweetened flavors. You might also add a little **Everly drink mix powder** or **Stur drink enhancer liquid**; these are both a safe way to make club soda taste like soda pop. Carbonated beverages give some people heartburn or flatulence, but hey, any port in a storm.

Tea and coffee help fill you up and they are unlimited on P2. **Loose-leaf green tea** is a modest appetite suppressant, due to its catechins. Unfortunately, you'd need to drink 8-10 cups of regular-strength, loose leaf green tea to get the full appetite suppressant effect. You may find ***Pique Green Tea Crystals*** helpful for hunger. The catechins in this concentrated, powdered green tea help manage grehlin, the hormone that signals hunger. Pique comes in individual serving packets that dilute well in either hot or cold water, which is a nice feature. You might try half a packet the first few times you use Pique; some patients have found that a full packet of concentrated green tea causes them mild nausea.

Fiber

Glucomannan (konjac root powder) is fiber that creates a gel when dissolved in warm water. You can drink that gel, which is quite filling. Konjac root powder is the same ingredient used in **shirataki noodles**. There's an entire section on uses for shirataki noodles, called "A Course in Miracle Noodles."

Glucomannan comes as a fine powder, so you can also **use as you'd use cornstarch** — to thicken a sauce or make a coating stick to something you're baking. No matter what form it takes, glucomannan is about bulking your food and drink up with very few calories. When adding indigestible fiber to your diet, be sure to drink extra water to prevent constipation (although some people experience the opposite effect).

Fiber also supports the health of your microbiome, which is quite relevant to weight loss. There are a vast number of bacterial cells in our microbiome. We are rapidly learning how microbiome health influences our metabolism and perhaps even determines it.

Fiber is also useful for weight loss because it has the potential to reduce the toxins that end up in our microbiome. Here's how: About 90% of the bile secreted by our liver is re-absorbed by the gut. That bile may contain toxins the body has been storing in fat. When we eat fiber, it binds to the bile, making it less toxic. Thus, fewer toxicants make it to our gut, which is good news for cultivating a healthy metabolism.

PGX Fiber is made of konjac root powder. Like glucomannan, you pour PGX fiber into warm water and drink it to help combat hunger. One 'pro' in favor of PGX is that it comes packaged in individual tubes and liquid capsules, for travel, if you prefer that to a scoop. One 'con' is that those tubes contain granules that are larger than glucomannan powder, so they don't dissolve as easily as glucomannan does.

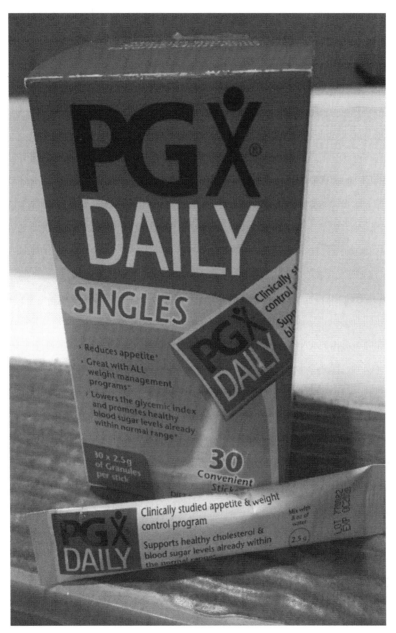

Photo: Dana Falk

PGX Fiber = glucomannan powder = shirataki noodles. All are forms of the fibrous konjac root, which is fine for HCG.

These products can be a terrific help with pushing through hunger, but one drawback to any product made with konjac root is that the high fiber content may constipate you. If you plan to weigh yourself in the morning and want to see the lowest possible number on the scale, don't take glucomannan late the night before. Your Number One concern may be hunger, but your weight will be up until you've enjoyed a Number Two.

Protein

There are several forms of concentrated protein that are useful for pushing through hunger. A high quality **whey protein isolate powder** does a crazy good job of creating satiety. It does have calories, but when blended with coffee and ice cubes, you've got a nice, big **latte shake** for those 100 or so calories. Even plain, unflavored whey protein powder tastes reasonably good. You can doll it up with a few shakes of **ground cinnamon** if you like. Higher quality cinnamon has a naturally sweet, floral taste.

For people who are lactose intolerant, **unflavored Egg White Protein Powder** is a better choice than whey protein would be. Unlike unflavored whey protein, though, it's quite difficult to disguise the flavor. For some, unflavored egg white protein tastes like an angora sweater at the bottom of the hamper. It's possible to make it taste good if you have cocoa powder or matcha powder, though. You might consider buying *flavored* egg white protein powder if you plan to use it on HCG — just be certain it has no sugar or artificial sweeteners. *Paleo Protein* and *Jay Robb* are both safe choices, but anything made with an alternative natural sweetener like stevia, xylitol, erythritol or monk fruit extract would be fine.

A scoop of **collagen peptide powder** isn't as filling as whey or egg white protein is, but it has fewer calories than they do and it **makes drinks creamy** when blended. It's far better for you than milk is when on HCG, so **try collagen blended in your coffee** if you need something creamy. Collagen also provides structure to grain-free baked goods, so mess around with it if you're trying to figure out to make some recipe **chewier, less fluffy or less crumbly.** Most of your baking will be after HCG, of course, but keep collagen peptide powder in your bag of tricks.

Another trick for pushing through hunger is to pour a scoop of collagen powder directly into your mouth. As it dissolves on your tongue, the collagen becomes chewy; it's neutral in flavor and kind of pleasing! A bit of 'collagen mouth taffy' is a weird hack, but it'd be a good name for an indie band and it may help push through hunger.

If you find you're terribly hungry after eating all your calories for the day, and you truly need more food, try eating more of a lean protein. Eat a **few extra prawns, another Greek meatball, a few slices of turkey breast or spoonfuls of your curried chicken salad.** Protein is substantial, it causes less insulin response than carbs do and it's unlikely to make you crave sweets.

Gum

For some people, chewing gum reduces appetite. Keep an eye out for your individual response, though: for a few people, chewing gum increases appetite. *Spry gum, PuR gum and XyliChew* are all made with alternative natural sweeteners, so they are more safe for HCG than sugar-free gums with aspartame, sucralose or saccharine are. All three of these brands have some interesting flavors, like green tea, cinnamon and chocolate mint, as well as the old school pink bubble gum and peppermint flavors.

Salt

One trick you might try to push through hunger is to place about 1/4 teaspoon of kosher salt in the middle of their tongue. *Allow the salt to dissolve to a liquid*, then swallow it. **Diamond Crystal kosher salt** is an especially good choice, since it's so mild in flavor.

This hack generally makes hunger pangs subside for 30-45 minutes, which is long enough for you to fall asleep without needing an after-dinner snack. Some people use the salt trick to decrease the number of times they eat each day, thus reducing the number of times they have an insulin response. It's a little creepy how well this trick works.

People in ketosis (like those on HCG) often need more salt than usual, due to electrolyte depletion. Unless you've been advised by a healthcare provider to eat low sodium, the salt trick should be useful at this time.

Use your evening routine

If you're hungry at night, try kicking into your evening clean-up routine: brush your teeth, floss, take out your contacts. If you have a bite guard or a retainer that goes in your mouth, clean it and put it in. If you have a skin regimen, a hair conditioning practice, supplements to take, tend to all of that. Scrape those rough heels, trim, tweeze. Symbolically, you are shifting focus from the "eating portion of the day" to the post-eating portion. Although this is purely symbolic, and you could certainly eat again after you have flossed, most people find that the change of focus to evening hygiene does distract them from food.

Go to bed early

Even with the HCG hormone reducing your appetite and a variety of tricks for pushing though, you are likely to feel hungry. Here's a strategy we learned from a patient: she said that when she had reached her calorie limit for the day, she put herself to bed, even if it was 7:00pm. What a simple, elegant solution!

Declare yourself done eating for the day once you head off to bed. Use a boring book or podcast to help you fall asleep. Listen to vocals or spoken-word in a language you don't understand, which can be very soothing. Don't bring work to bed or you'll still be alert enough to feel your hunger. Some people find that a warm bath or shower helps them feel sleepy. There are some other solo activities that tend to make people feel sleepy.

Clever Strategies for P2 Cooking

Having special equipment can be a big help to your cooking. The items below are not kitchen essentials by any means, but they may expand your repertoire while on P2, which is nice when you have limited options. Of course, these are all tools you could use well beyond your HCG round, when you will still be looking for tasty, healthy meal prep ideas but have more ingredients and calories to work with.

Kitchen tools expand your repertoire

<u>Non-stick waffle iron</u>

Make yourself a **waffle omelet!** First the rationale, then the recipe. The original HCG protocol says you may eat a whole egg if you eat it with the whites of three additional eggs. We find that eating a whole egg about once a week (without all that extra egg white) is perfectly fine for patients. It's probably better actually, since we now know that unusually high protein consumption (like four egg whites at one sitting) would trigger an insulin response. You're better off just having an occasional whole egg, in our opinion. Add one additional egg white if you wish, to give your omelet more bulk.

How much would an omelette in the shape of a waffle improve your mood when you've been eating like a rabbit? Right, it probably wouldn't hurt.

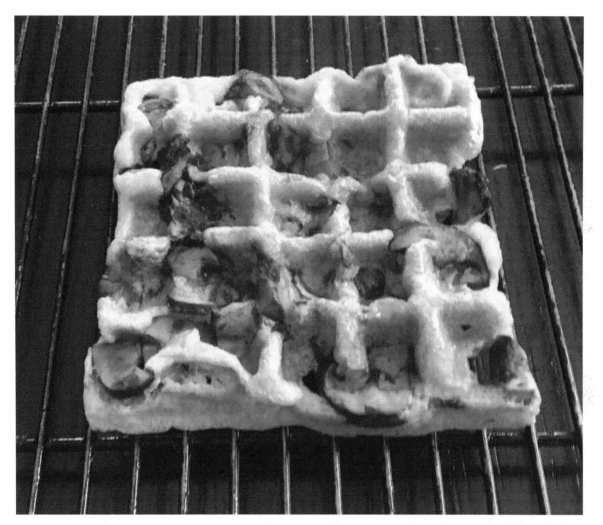

Photo: Dana Falk

Crimini mushrooms, salt and one egg are cooked in a Belgian waffle maker on medium heat to make a waffle omelet. It's not really a waffle but it's fun. Use medium-low heat if you don't want the egg to brown.

Waffle Omelet

Set your waffle iron to the low or medium-low heat.

Lightly beat one egg, with an additional egg white if you'd like (but your omelet will taste richer without it).

Add 1/8 tsp kosher salt and a dash of grated nutmeg. That's your blank canvas.

Now add flavor to that blank canvas, if you wish.

Mix-in ideas: roasted cherry tomatoes, garlic spinach, crab meat, leftover meatloaf crumbles, jalapeños, roasted bell pepper, crawfish, mushrooms sautéed in fat-free chicken broth, basil, fresh thyme, leftover pork tenderloin with curry powder, small amount of caramelized onion, small amount of artichoke heart, sambal olek (chili paste), salsa verde, baked eggplant, roasted zucchini, leftover chicken.

Pour the egg into one section of your waffle iron, then immediately disperse your mix-in ingredients on top.

Close the waffle iron and let it run its full cycle on low heat.

Remove your waffle omelet by using two forks to loosen the edges. Transfer to a rack rather than a plate, so it can rest a moment without the steam making it soggy.

You can amuse yourself by cooking other things in your waffle iron, too. A **portobello mushroom** would char well, as would **calamari or octopus, sliced eggplant, a chicken or turkey breast pounded thin or slices of lemon.** Roasted lemon gives you super delicious juice you can squeeze onto meat, seafood or veggies and into dressings and marinades.

Digital meat thermometer

You'll notice we often write that some meat or fish is done when it reaches a particular internal temperature. Not knowing how thick your cuts are, how big a piece you're cooking, whether you've chosen to bake, broil, grill or sous vide means that suggesting an internal temperature is the best guidance we can provide about when your food will be done.

If you don't already own an instant read, digital meat thermometer, you'll find it a worthy investment at about $15-$20. The basic version has a probe attached to a long handle with the digital readout. Stick the probe into the thickest part of the meat or fish while it's still cooking and you get a status report. There are also fancier digital food thermometers that have a long cord between the probe and the readout, so the probe may be inside a hot oven and the readout on you kitchen counter. You insert the probe in the uncooked food, set the readout to your desired temperature and it will beep when the food reaches that number. These cost a bit more, of course.

If you love to cook, a digital food thermometer will be useful well beyond your time on HCG.

Slow cooker or crockpot

A slow cooker maximizes the flavors you have to work with because they have time to mingle. It's great for **stewing lean meats with broth** to make them more tender, or making a **gumbo** or **chili** out of leftover veggies, meat or seafood and Cajun spices.

Because flavors develop in a slow cooker, you could make a batch of **collard greens** taste good with a small amount of onion and garlic (which are higher carb ingredients) and still get those great flavors. Add some bones and some apple cider vinegar or hot sauce and you've got collards.

A canned **chicken broth that's had fennel simmering in it** all day is on another plane from that same broth straight out of the can. Fennel-infused chicken broth then becomes your stir fry liquid or soup base. Imagine **asparagus soup** made by pureeing that fennel-infused broth, cooked asparagus and smoked maldon salt in the blender.

Do turkey breast + jalapeño + whole allspice + miracle noodles + the bones of a rotisserie chicken make a nice **turkey noodle soup** after three hours together in a slow cooker? Find out. (Spoiler alert: they do.)

Slow Cooker Chili

Recipe contributed by Robin Lesh

This recipe makes quite a large batch of chili, 16 servings. Since this dish is an ideal way to use leftover bits of meat and vegetables, feel free to make a smaller batch — whatever you have enough ingredients on hand for. Grinding your own turkey breast or other protein enables you to control the fat content and to disperse the flavor.

3 cups (two 12 oz cans) fire roasted, diced tomatoes, including liquid

One 8 oz can diced, mild green chiles

3 lbs ground turkey or other P2 meat, ground in food processor

4 cups fat free chicken broth

4 cups chopped celery

3 medium zucchini, chopped roughly

3 cups white or crimini mushrooms, quartered

2 cups sliced cabbage

1/2 tsp sea salt

Up to 3/4 tsp each (to taste): cayenne, cumin

Optional:

Other leftover P2 veggies, such as bell peppers, eggplant, turnip

Up to 1/2 tsp Hatch chili powder

Up to 2 cloves garlic

Up to 1/2 tsp onion powder

Up to 3 dashes worcestershire sauce

1 bay leaf

— Place all ingredients in slow cooker. Simmer 6-8 hours on high if you've used some raw meat in your chili. Done at 4-5 hours if you've used all cooked meat.

— If time allows, allow chili to rest overnight in the refrigerator. This will deepen flavors.

— Portion some of the chili into small containers to freeze for quick meals.

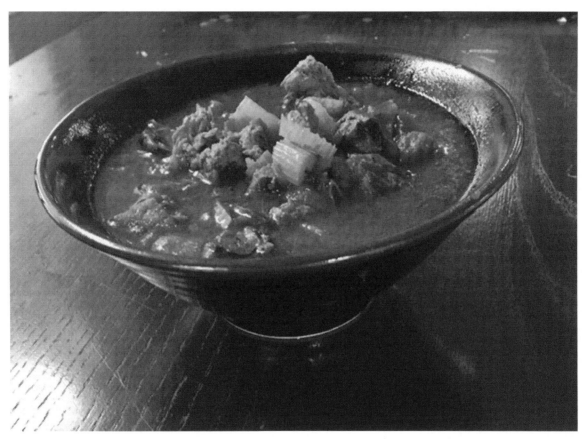

Photo: Dana Falk

Slow cooker chili made with raw ground turkey and leftover cooked beef. This rendition has no zucchini (hate it) extra celery (love it) and a mildly spicy broth. Use whatever you've got!

Flat BBQ skewers

It's much easier to get char on your grilled food when the pieces of meat and vegetables don't twirl on round skewers. *Inspired Stainless Steel Skewers* come six to a box and are inexpensive.

Grilling over charcoal is a great way to make it through HCG with flavorful food, but you can also get some char on a gas grill, in a cast iron pan, over an open flame or even on a cookie sheet at high heat.

Here's a nice use for flat BBQ skewers: Make an Afghani yogurt marinade for your protein of choice, let sit overnight, wipe yogurt off, then grill the following day. The basic recipe is called **Kebab e Murgh**. On HCG, this may be accomplished with chicken breast (it's usually made with thighs) with goat meat (it's usually done with lamb) with swordfish or other firm fish, with bison and even with firm veggies like cauliflower.

You can eat chicken thigh and lamb while on HCG, but you wouldn't be able to have much of it. We suggest that you consider making a slightly less traditional version of kebab e murgh, using chicken breast, so you can eat more of it.

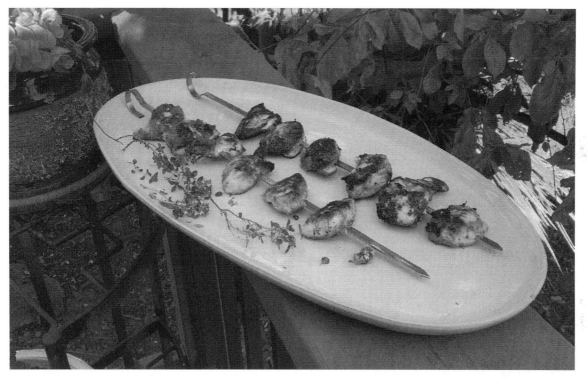

Photo: Dana Falk

Kebab e murgh is one of many dishes made better by flat BBQ skewers. This chicken breast was in a yogurt marinade overnight. It has taken on the yellow-orange color of the tumeric, the tang of the yogurt and the woodsy flavor of the fresh thyme.

Kebab e Murgh
Afghani yogurt-marinated shish-kebab

Allow to marinate at least six hours in the fridge before grilling. The yogurt tenderizes and flavors the kebabs but is wiped off before grilling. The yogurt should be enough to marinate at least 2.5 pounds of meat.

2-3 pounds meat, fish or protein of choice
Suggestions: chicken breast, goat, cauliflower, eggplant, swordfish, halibut, prawns

2 cups plain, nonfat yogurt
The juice of 1/2 medium lemon (save that half lemon)
1 tsp fresh garlic, grated
1 tsp fresh ginger, grated

1/2 tsp ground coriander
1/2 tsp cumin
Not everyone likes cumin and coriander. These are traditional, but substitute 1 tsp curry powder (total) if you prefer.

1/2 tsp paprika or sumac (paprika is traditional)
1 tsp tumeric
1 tsp sea salt
1/4 cup chopped flat leaf parsley, cilantro or mint.

Optional: 2 tsp granulated alternative natural sweetener or 1 tbs All-u-lose Honey syrup. Not traditional for murgh, but balances the spices nicely.

— Cut your meat, fish or veggies into 2 inch chunks. Set aside.

— Combine ingredients above in a non-metal bowl or pan. Tumeric and paprika are likely to stain your bowl if you use plastic, so glass is your best bet.

— Roughly chop the lemon half you have juiced and add to mixture.

— Once spices are well incorporated in yogurt, add your kebab meat/fish/veg to the marinade. Stir to assure all are coated in yogurt.

— Cover and refrigerate 6-24 hours.

— When ready to cook, heat grill surface to medium high.

— Remove meat/fish/veg from marinade and lightly wipe yogurt off each piece, using paper towels. It's not important they be totally dry, just wipe them the best you can.

— Place meat/fish/veg on your flat skewers, with 1/4 inch between pieces for best browning. If you are making more than one kind of kebab (let's say some are chicken, some are fish) place only one kind of protein on each skewer, since they will cook for different lengths of time.

— Place your skewers on hot grill, cast iron pan, etc. Allow to char well on one side before turning.

— Grill on second side to desired doneness and remove from heat. Use a fork to slide the cooked kebabs off their skewers.

— Garnish with more fresh herbs and enjoy.

Spiralizer

A spiralizer enables you to turn a crank and produce long strings of vegetables. **Zucchini and other summer squash** put through a spiralizer resemble noodles. Cooking them just briefly in heavily salted boiling water provides a bed for whatever protein you're making. Veggies with solid structure, like **cucumbers and chayote squash**, go through a spiralizer beautifully. Long, curly strands of cucumber with a vinaigrette of rice vinegar, MCT oil, lime juice and a sweetener like Swerve makes a **tangy, curly cucumber salad** that's even better when it's been in the fridge for at least an hour.

Technically, you can use a spiralizer on hollow veggies like bell pepper, but it requires more patience and some experimenting with the various blades. For example, using a spiralizer on a bell pepper with a slicing disk would render super thin, julienne strips.

A spiralizer gives you an appealing way to present a salad or side dish to others while you're on P2, but it's practical, too: **thinly sliced veggies are easier to make tasty** with a dressing or vinaigrette than thick-cut ones are. Spiralizers are inexpensive; it's finding a place to store them that's a drag. That would be a good problem for you to have when you're down a size, wouldn't it?

Cast iron pan

Getting food to brown without using oil in the pan is a bitch. Your best bet will be to use either a cast iron pan or a panini grill (below). Cast iron pans are reasonably priced if you avoid the ones that are enameled. You may find a cast iron pan in thrift store, too, though these usually require some rehabilitation.

The trick is to pre-heat a cast iron thoroughly before you put food in it. Some people heat it at medium-high for 2-3 minutes, others put it in the oven for 20 minutes. Cast iron retains heat extremely well, but it takes time to get there. One you've got a hot cast iron pan, it's your best chance at getting some color on meat and veggies.

To care for a cast iron pan, avoid cooking anything acidic. No tomatoes, vinegar or citrus juice in your stir fry Never scrub with soap or put through the dishwasher. Use salt and warm water as your abrasive.

Panini grill

A panini grill enables you to grill things on both sides at the same time. One P2 trick is to make a **"sandwich" with slices of turkey meat on the outside**, as the bread. Inside could be a cooked egg, some pesto, mushrooms and arugula. If you like alfalfa sprouts, these help bulk out any sandwich and are surprisingly filling. As a Tier 1 veggie, you could eat an awful big heap of alfalfa sprouts.

Asparagus cooked on a panini grill is genius, but you'll need to blanch it first (boil briefly) so that you can be sure it cooks through. Ditto for **eggplant and green beans or Chinese long beans. Raw calamari and prawns** you can cook on a panini grill without prepping.

Playing with a panini grill can be fun. What if you were to shred Brussels sprouts and pile those on a panini grill? Once they are charred you'd remove them from the grill and toss in a light dressing. You'd have created a **warm Brussels sprout salad**.

Fancy restaurants sometimes serve a **grilled Caesar salad**; there's no reason you couldn't slice a head of romaine lettuce in half, char it on the panini grill, then remove and dress it. You can't make classic Caesar dressing on HCG because it has oily anchovies, but you could substitute smoked trout or some other fish in your Caesar dressing. You could also make your go-to MCT "honey mustard" vinaigrette, which would be great on grilled romaine. You could also use your one whole egg for the week, hard boil it and chop it on top of the grilled Caesar.

Food dehydrator

If you're feeling ambitious, you can make yourself **chewy meat jerky or crispy dried vegetable chips** for trail snacks in a food dehydrator. This is a big lug of a machine, but do consider getting one because (a) it can increase your snack repertoire while on HCG and (b) it's mighty fun beyond HCG. People make dog treats, dried fruit, yogurt...there are a ton of interesting ways to use a food dehydrator.

There's an entire section on homemade jerky under "Quick Bite Ideas." The short version is this: most pre-packaged jerky has sugar. You can dehydrate jerky that is tailored to your tastes (spicy, sweet, salty) and is sugar-free.

Silicone molds

If you decide to use unflavored gelatin to make **chewy, gummy desserts**, silicone molds make them look fancy. There are molds in the shape of Swedish fish and gummy bears and dinosaurs. There are molds in the shape of small, individual squares to help your portion your treats. Making gummy desserts is highly recommended on Phase 2, and silicone molds make it look like you've accomplished something good enough to share.

Check out the section "Quick Bite Ideas" for a bunch more on using unflavored gelatin to make chewy desserts. You will not be able to buy most sugar-free, boxed gelatin desserts on the market and just add boiling water. At this writing, sugar free gelatin is usually made with artificial sweeteners, not with alternative natural sweeteners. You'll probably need to engineer these gummy desserts yourself, because artificial sweeteners may stall your weight loss.

<u>Popsicle molds</u>

A set of popsicle molds gives so much bang for the buck. Fun, inexpensive and available in a wild variety of shapes, you will appreciate this investment when you're craving a little treat.

Once you have the molds, blend iced tea and a little fruit to create a batch of **gourmet popsicles**. Just a tiny bit of fruit makes a big difference to the flavor.

<u>Here are a few flavor combinations for your popsicles:</u>

Rhubarb or orange spice tea with a little frozen strawberry blended in

Blackberry sage tea with a few real blackberries blended in

Tazo cucumber tea + pureed cucumber + watermelon blended in

Earl grey tea + lemon blended in

Hibiscus tea + fresh raspberries blended in

If you are not eating fruit at all on P2, use any of the drinks or drink mixes made with stevia, erythritol, xylitol, allulose or monk fruit. Everly, Bai and Ultima drinks are flavorful and safe for P2, for most people.

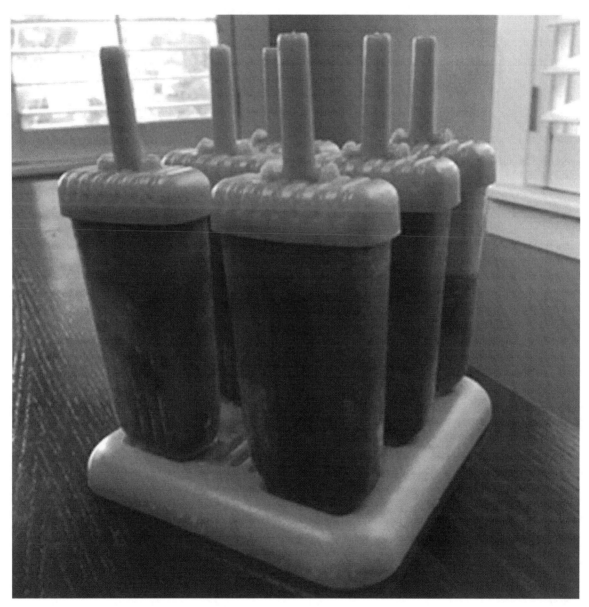

Photo: Dana Falk

Hibiscus iced tea with stevia glycerite becomes a snack when blended with a few raspberries and frozen into popsicle molds.

Ingredients that Impart Lots of Flavor

Chicken broth	Chicken carcass	Crustacean shells	Mushroom broth
Coconut aminos	Tamari	Fish sauce	Clam juice
Apple cider vinegar	Coconut vinegar	Rice Vinegar (plain)	Meyer lemon
Star anise	Clove	Allspice	Chinese five spice
Fresh mint	Fresh celery leaves	Fresh basil	Fresh thyme
Citrus zest or pith	Fennel bulb	Caper berries	Fenugreek
Garam masala	Curry powder	Red pepper flakes	Smoked paprika
Fresh ginger	Galanga (young ginger)	Kaffir lime leaves	Lemongrass
Wasabi	Tumeric root	Hot sauce	Starfruit
Kim chee	Dried seaweed (nori) sheets	Unsweetened cocoa	Matcha powder
Espresso powder	Hibiscus tea	Vanilla beans	Cinnamon sticks, cinnamon tea

All of these ingredients are potent in flavor with very few calories, so they can be helpful for cooking on Phase 2. If you can find just a few on the list that please you, exploit them to prevent boredom.

— **Fresh ginger** is delicious grated directly into your water bottle.

— A dash of **rice vinegar or coconut vinegar** would make stir fry taste brighter.

— **Shredded nori (seaweed)** makes egg taste more savory and interesting.

— Blending your vanilla whey protein shake with **crushed green tea ice cubes** rather than plain water ice cubes creates sophisticated flavor.

— A small amount of **grated horseradish root or wasabi root** brings a bitter heat that's entirely different from making something spicy using hot peppers. Try either of them on plain vegetable dishes, bland shirataki noodles, inside meat roll ups or sushi rolls.

Tomatillos are on Tier 2; they are surprisingly good for HCG, given how much character they bring to any dish. Similar in flavor to tomatillos are **green tomatoes**, which are also on Tier 2. In both cases, you can fire roast them and make a salsa verde. You can dice them and use in a slow cooker dish with meat. If given enough time, they break down into a sour, thick sauce that brings a Mexican (tomatillo) or Southern (green tomato) flavor palette to any dish.

Meyer lemons warrant special mention because there's so much you can do with them. They are a hybrid fruit that has more carbohydrate than standard lemons do, but we think they're worth it in small quantities. Normally, lemons are sharply acidic; fantastic for bringing brightness to foods but too sour to use in many dishes. Meyer lemons they have a more mellow, more dimensional flavor than standard lemons do; moderately bitter, moderately sour, slightly sweet. With a less intense flavor profile and a slightly softer rind, Meyer lemons are tremendously versatile.

You can **pulverize a *whole* Meyer lemon** — peel, pith, fruit and all. Cut it in half, remove the seeds, microwave for 15 seconds and chuck the lemon halves into your food processor. The resulting **Meyer lemon puree** can be used to bring big flavor to a variety off things: it's fantastic on cooked spinach or asparagus, makes a **flavorful topping to roast with fish and shellfish**, makes a yummy salad dressing or marinade.

Pureed Meyer lemon is a sophisticated **addition to your pitcher of iced tea**. It turns your vanilla protein mug cake into a **lemon mug cake** and turns plain gelatin squares into tangy, **gummy lemonade squares**. Boost your foodie credentials.

Twenty-Two Techniques that Create Flavor

1. Get your paws on some high quality salt

There's **lavender fleur de sel, applewood smoked salt, smoked maldon flakes, rosemary salt,**...so much to choose from that tastes better than table salt. There's even smoked black pepper! You can salt your food as liberally as you'd like on HCG. In fact, being in ketosis tends to deplete people of their sodium. You may be surprised by how nothing more than high-quality salt enhances flavor. If you don't want to mess with fancy salts, get some very mild kosher salt, such as ***Diamond Crystal*** salt. Because it's not intensely salty, you have some room for error. Diamond Crystal is great for just making whatever you're cooking taste a bit better.

If you do have energy for finding specialty salts and such, find an import store in your town or take to the internet. Finding **Mediterranean, Middle Eastern and African spice mixes** may inspire you. The same is true for **English teas.** Think you've tasted cinnamon? Try **Vietnamese ground cinnamon**; it will restore your faith in humanity. With its sweet, floral notes, try it in your coffee grounds instead of adding sweetener to your cup. Cinnamon works for both sweet and savory dishes, so try it on pork tenderloin, your slow cooker chicken tinga and your chocolate whey protein shake.

Salt will work harder for you if you give it some time with the foods you're seasoning before cooking them. If you plan to cook plain turkey breast, which can be dry, salting the meat an hour before you will cook it and returning it to the fridge will make the finished turkey more flavorful. If you're making broccoli, blanch briefly in very salty boiling water, then drain before doing a stir fry. Salt gives always you a running start to flavor.

2. Try citrus rind and membranes

Oranges, tangerines, pomelo and some other citrus fruits are too high in carbs for us to recommend eating the whole fruit while on HCG, but the bitter rind, with its **oily zest** on the outside and its **bitter white pith** on the inside is tremendously useful. So are the tough **segment membranes** that divide the sweet juicy segments from one another. Basically, if you were to completely juice an orange, so that what's left is a little dry pulp, segment membranes and the rind, *that is what's useful* for HCG cooking.

Now you have a bitter and tangy ingredient to work with. It's complex and intense and works for both sweet and savory dishes. For example, soaking any **citrus rind in warm water** will give you a flavor infusion. That creates a delicious citrus-infused water you could use for making **iced tea, a gelatin dessert, a brine for seafood or a braising liquid for chicken or fish. Baking fish** alongside the empty half of a lime or grapefruit you have already squeezed on the flesh adds a layer of flavor, too.

If it's too hard for you to have sweet citrus in the house and only use the rind, don't do it. But if you can give away the juice or stick it in the freezer for later, you've got some amazing iced tea in your future.

3. Roast citrus slices

If you **slice lemons very thinly** you can roast them with your veggies or slow cook them with your meat to really punch up the flavor. The juice of a raw lemon can be sharp and acidic, but roasting thin slices caramelizes them, rendering more mellow flavor. For example, try making **lemon roasted Brussels sprouts**.

Lemon Roasted Brussels Sprouts

1 pound fresh Brussels Sprouts
1/2 tsp good quality salt
1 large lemon
Optional: 1 tbs fresh chopped thyme or herb of choice

— Preheat oven to 400° F

— Trim the hard ends from 1 pound of Brussels sprouts.

— Cut the sprouts in half lengthwise and place in a single layer on a baking sheet. If you have any humongous sprouts, quarter them.

— Cut lemon in half. Place one of the halves cut side down on baking sheet.

— Slice the other lemon half into very thin slices. Arrange the slices on the baking sheet with the cut sprouts.

— If using fresh herbs, chop roughly and add to sprouts. Thyme is excellent with this dish.

— Toss the cut sprouts and herbs in the best salt you've got.

— Roast sprouts in 400° F oven for 15-17 minutes, rotating the baking tray and shaking it to toss the sprouts at the 10 minute mark.

TIP: Because you aren't using oil, the sprouts won't brown much, so it can be difficult to tell when they're done. Poke a sharp knife into one of the larger sprouts at 15 minutes to see whether it has cooked through. Continue roasting if you'd like them more tender.

— The finished sprouts will have a subtle roasted lemon flavor from the thin slices cooking with them. (Save the slices and puree them for another dish, if you'd like.)

— If you want more pronounced lemon flavor, squeeze the juice of the half lemon that has roasted on the pan. (If not, save that for another dish. It's gold.)

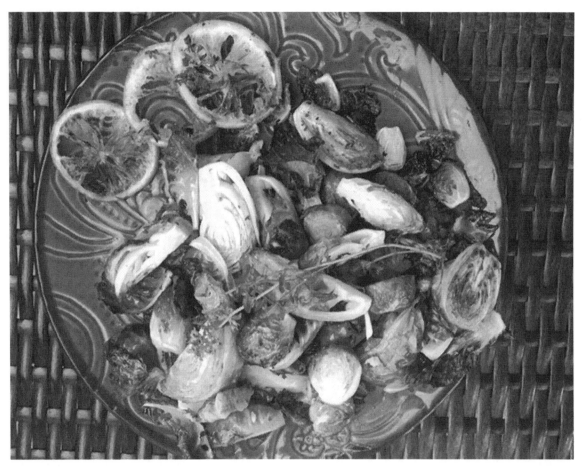

Photo: Dana Falk

Brussels sprouts roasted at 400° with fresh thyme and a squeeze of roasted lemon taste really good. These are a Tier 3 veggie so this dish would be considered a large a portion, but Brussels sprouts are quite filling.

Another trick with citrus is to add thin slices to a slow cooker dish. For example, you could toss chicken breast and lemon slices into a slow cooker. If the lemons have been sliced thinly enough and cooked long enough, they will essentially melt into the dish and you needn't remove them. You'd then have a **slow cooker lemon chicken**. Meyer lemons are less sour and are recommended for any dish in which the slices stay in. Try slow cooker lemon chicken over **cauliflower rice**.

4. For moistness and flavor, bake in packets

Parchment paper, banana leaves, tin foil and poultry roasting bags will all help you accomplish the same thing: you can stuff them full of goodies to create a **baking packet**. Inside of that packet, flavor and moistness are maximized. For example, **halibut baked with fresh ginger and bok choy in a foil packet** will turn out more moist and flavorful than halibut prepared on a cookie sheet, separately from the veggies will. Not only that, your entire meal is ready at once and clean-up is practically non-existent.

A classic preparation of baking packets is in parchment paper, called *en papillote* in French and Spanish cooking. If you'd like to bake your packets in banana leaves or lotus leaves, you can often find them in the freezer section of East Asian or Southeast Asian markets. The leaves themselves impart flavor to the dish in a way that foil and parchment cannot.

To create a baking packet, choose the flavors you want to mingle; perhaps a protein, some fresh herbs or spices and a veggie.

Examples of flavors you might build together in a baking packet:

— **Prawns with broccoli rabe and garlic**

— **Cornish hen with kale and tarragon**

— **Pork tenderloin with cabbage and sage**

— **Bison steak with bell peppers and cherry tomato**

— **Codfish with collard greens and Anaheim peppers**

— **Lobster with Swiss chard and lemongrass**

— **Chicken breast with zucchini and basil**

— **Lamb sirloin with turnips and harissa spice**

DANA FALK, PH.D. & KELSEY KLAUSMEYER, N.D.

Parchment baking packet (*en papillote*)

— Tear off about 16 inches of parchment paper or aluminum foil. Place it on a cookie sheet and have the cookie sheet facing you horizontally, so it's wide, left to right.

— Arrange the protein and veggies loosely, in the middle of the paper, intermingling with each other. If using aromatics (ginger, garlic, lemongrass, rosemary, etc.) be sure these are distributed throughout; they lend flavor but will not be eaten.

— Roll the paper with food inside horizontally, so you end up with long, open ends. The food is placed in the middle, so these ends should be empty.

— Tuck those empty ends *beneath* the packet (on the seam side) to form a closed packet.

— You'll now have a baking packet seam side down on a cookie sheet, ready to go in the oven. (Do *not* poke vent holes on top; leave it sealed.)

— Bake packets at 400° F and monitor doneness by checking with a meat thermometer. You can poke the thermometer right through the packet.

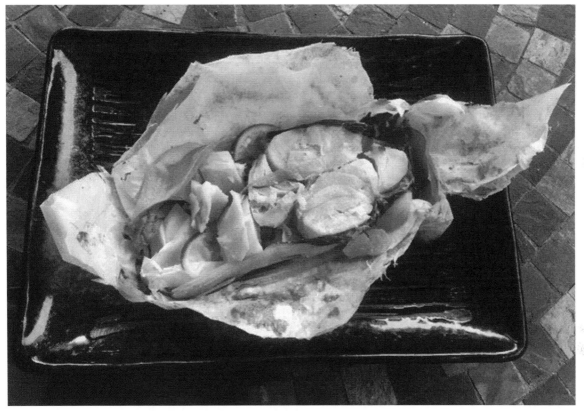

Photo: Dana Falk

Chunks of cod, baby bok choy, lime and ginger go into a parchment packet with a splash of fish sauce. After 25 minutes in a 400 degree oven, the packet is snipped open along the top. The cod and bok choy now taste like lime and ginger! This packet was cooked longer than needed; find your favorite fillings and their ideal cook time together.

— Venison calls for an internal temp of 120° F (rare) to 135° F (medium rare).

— Cod and pork tenderloin are considered done at an internal temperature of 145° F.

— Lamb is usually cooked to 145° F - 155° F.

— Bison is considered done at 160° F.

— White meat turkey is considered done at 165° F.

— Lobster would be ready at 160° F to 175° F.

— Cornish hens would be cooked to an internal temp of 180° F.

You can of course cook your proteins to the doneness you most enjoy. Since there's a different internal temperature associated with each protein at rare/medium rare/medium and beyond, you might prefer to look up the recommended temperature for what you're cooking. Remember that super lean meats quickly become chewy at higher internal temps, so if you're on the fence between medium rare and medium, try medium rare first.

5. Skillet cooking with lid creates a sauce

Not every meal while you're on HCG is likely to be a masterpiece; sometimes you'll just need a way to make whatever you have taste as good as possible. One technique for creating flavor is to cook in a skillet with the lid *on*, to create a sauce. Often we leave the lid off, to make skillet foods as crisp as possible, but for HCG cooking we need a Plan B. We won't be using oil, so making things crisp is not usually within reach.

To create a dish with its own sauce, sauté your dish about halfway way through without a lid. With a few minutes of cook time remaining, add a tiny bit of liquid: water, broth, vinegar, tea, coconut aminos, hot sauce, etc. Now complete the cooking with the lid on; this will render your finished dish a little saucier, with flavors better dispersed.

For example, mushrooms sautéed in broth + a little canned tomato + liquid added halfway through and the lid on = **a light mushroom sauce** you could use as a **topping for**

eggs, beef, spinach, or as the base of a soup. If you were to cook beef in a skillet with mushrooms and canned tomato, lid on, you'd have **savory beef with mushroom** as an entree that has made its own sauce. This should be fairly satisfying on its own or would be good eaten over cauliflower rice or greens.

6. Make potent sauces, then use just a little

The more potent a sauce is, the less of it you'll need to create flavor. Since you'll have so few calories to work with on HCG, being able to sauce things lightly and still have flavor to enjoy helps your calorie count for the day.

For example, if you've made a batch of chicken mole in your slow cooker, put the finished chicken in a colander with a container beneath it to catch the sauce. **Drain the chicken thoroughly but save that mole sauce** for other dishes. The chicken meat that was cooking for hours in mole sauce for hours will *already* have tons of flavor. You can drain it completely and it will still be delicious. Draining off the sauce reduces your per-serving calories for the dish.

The leftover mole sauce will be very potent, tasting of both chicken and mole. You can spoon it over other meat dishes, use it as a dipping sauce or condiment. You may also use it as the start of a second batch of chicken mole in the slow cooker. This time, the dish will take nearly no time to prepare, since you'd simply be placing raw meat into finished sauce and firing up the slow cooker.

7. Use high heat to develop flavor and color

Climb to the top kitchen cabinet for your panini grill, rescue your George Foreman grill from the garage, clean and season the cast iron pan you have avoided. Any time you can apply high heat to food, you generate flavor. Some of the suggestions here are foods we don't ordinarily cook over direct high heat, but the goal is just to render some flavor: smoky, browned, even slightly burned are welcomed while on HCG.

Broiling white fish gives it some color. Roasting veggies makes them sweeter. For example, dense, crunchy **fennel becomes sweet**, tender and aromatic when roasted. Bland celery becomes slightly browned and more flavorful in the oven.

Charring food over direct heat makes flavor more smoky and dimensional. Think about how much better a **bell pepper** tastes when it's been **charred over a direct flame** and has developed blackened, blistered skin. Eggplant roasted over an open flame until charred, then pureed with lemon, salt and garlic becomes an HCG version of **babaganoush** (minus the traditional sesame tahini, which has high fat content).

If possible, cook meat and vegetables on a grill, grill pan or in a cast iron pan. Cast iron takes a while to heat through, so give it a running start in the oven for at least 20 minutes before you add ingredients. Grill pans should be pre-heated on the stove top; flick a little water on them to assure they're screaming hot before adding your ingredients.

If you have a gas stove, placing veggies directly on the flame requires you to pay close attention, but it imparts crazy good flavor. **Charring a pasilla or Anaheim pepper**, both of which are mild-medium spicy, gives you an amazing ingredient to work with. These may go **diced, on a taco salad or in a batch of chili**. They may be **pureed to sauce egg whites or fish.** They might be hollowed out and used to make **chile relleno** (fill with ground meat, spices, an egg white and bake). You could make a **spicy, smoky vinaigrette to dress a seared tuna steak or tuna salad**. You might use this vinaigrette to **dress cooked veggies** like broccoli, broccoli rabe, Swiss chard or cauliflower. That smoky vinaigrette could also be drizzled on your **grilled radicchio or grilled romaine**.

8. Blanch veggies and dress while warm

You know how German potato salad tastes best if you add the bacon dressing to the boiled potatoes while they are still warm? The same principle applies to making veggie salads full-flavored while on HCG. Dress blanched vegetables while still warm, then serve at room temp or chill for later.

Let's say you're making a **broccoli salad with basil-lime vinaigrette** for HCG Phase 2. Make a vinaigrette of lime juice, MCT oil, crushed basil leaves, a pinch of salt and a smidge of sweetener like Swerve (optional). Boil your broccoli florets briefly in very salty water, until bright green. Drain the broccoli thoroughly then toss it with your vinaigrette while it's still warm. Once the salad is at room temperature you can either serve it immediately or refrigerate for later. Either way, don't allow the blanched broccoli to cool completely before you dress it.

Another application of dressing veggies while warm: let's say you make a **spicy cauliflower salad** you plan to serve at room temperature. Use the same procedure as above, but make a spicy vinaigrette of apple cider vinegar, MCT oil, sweetener and either wasabi, hot mustard, Thai chiles or hot curry powder to add some heat. Cauliflower will absorb whatever flavors you introduce; even more so if you get that dressing on while it's still warm.

9. Try high quality flavor extracts

There are high-quality **natural flavor extracts** available online. These are not sweeteners and they do not contain alcohol. In addition to familiar flavors like banana, coconut, maple and almond, there are *savory* flavor extracts that may stimulate your creativity for P2 cooking. For example, there are natural extracts in cashew, corn, juniper, parmesan, violet, eucalyptus, graham cracker and pine smoke flavors. Be careful to buy extracts or natural flavoring, not flavored oils.

Some inspiration for your use of extracts: add a few drops of **rose extract** to your peach gelatin squares for an Indian or Persian flavor profile. Try a few drops of **juniper extract** in Zevia tonic water to emulate a gin and tonic. A few drops of **graham cracker flavor** in a Quest cinnamon crunch whey shake would taste very comforting. A few drops of **oak smoke or sassafras extract** in a marinade for beef jerky would make the flavor more complex. Try **rum flavor** in a sauce for shrimp or a coffee drink. There are a lot of potential uses for extract in the hands of creative cooks.

Online, www.BestFlavors.com is one option for high quality extracts. They also carry **flavor drops specifically for drinking water**, made with stevia. These come in a wider variety of flavors than you would find as prepared drinks.

10. Brine first

You can brine any meat, sturdy seafood or sturdy veggies. You can make a wet brine (submerge the food in salty water) or a dry brine (rub a salt only, or a salt + spice mix directly on the food). You let the raw food sit in this salty water or savory rub for at least an hour. There's a recipe below.

Brining maximizes flavor. With proteins, brining helps retain moisture, as well. The technique is a godsend for salvaging very lean meats, which benefit from any strategy that makes them more tender. We'll focus here on how to create a wet brine.

Basic Wet Brine

1/4 cup kosher salt + 4 cups water = basic wet brine.
Don't use table salt or your brine will be far too salty.

Stir to dissolve the salt in the water.

Recommended: add aromatics to your basic brine, like whole cardamom pods, whole cinnamon sticks, bay leaves, allspice, fresh fennel, Sichuan peppercorns, sliced jalapeños, fresh sage, garlic cloves, 1/4 onion or some citrus rind.

If you'd like a super long list of possible aromatics for your brine, skip ahead to the section called "Basic Refrigerator Pickles."

The aromatics you add to a wet brine will impart just a subtle flavor, unless you use a lot of them or you brine your food for a long time.

Optional: add 2 tbs Swerve alternative natural sweetener.
Salt + a little sweet = extra delicious results. Think kettle corn.

Time in wet brine:
30 minutes minimum * 1-2 hours is most common * overnight maximum

Fortunately, as little as 30 minutes in a wet brine can enhance the flavor of your food. In general, plan to brine foods at least one hour in the refrigerator.

Be sure to *thoroughly pat dry* anything you have soaked in a brine solution before you cook it, so it will not steam. Cook brined food at high heat: on a grill, in a cast iron pan on the stove or on a cookie sheet in the oven at 425 degrees.

If you enjoy cooking, you'll make good use of your brining experiments long after HCG.

11. Serve vegetables sliced thick, into "steaks"

It may sound bizarre, but there are high-end restaurants that serve **cauliflower steaks**. A whole cauliflower is sliced from top to stem, an inch or more thick. The florets should hold together, giving you a steak. That's then smoked, baked or grilled. Drizzle it with the sauce of your choice and you've got a meal for very few calories.

TIP: As a home cook, it's not a bad idea to give your cauliflower steak a running start with being cooked through before you grill it. We suggest brining a cauliflower steak, then microwaving it for 90 seconds before popping it into the oven or onto the grill. If the cauliflower doesn't turn out tender and a little creamy on the interior, you might give up on prematurely on this technique.

You may also experiment with the "steak technique" using a head of cabbage, a turnip, a large bunch of broccoli and any other HCG-friendly veggie that is dense enough for you to play with shape in this way. Cauliflower is the classic, though, because its tight structure helps it hold together and because it gets custardy when cooked properly.

12. Use onion as flavor base, not primary ingredient

Onions are sweet and delicious but they are pretty carby. If you peel an onion and quarter it, leaving the stem and root ends on, you can use it to **develop flavor in the base of your soup or stewing liquid** for its sweet, earthy flavor — then easily remove the whole thing, the way you would remove a bay leaf. While on HCG Phase 2, that's a better investment of your carbs and calories than eating sliced onions in a stir fry or chopped onions on chili would be.

If you want onion as an *ingredient*, consider cooking it low and slow to caramelize. The flavor of caramelized onion is so potent, so you can very little of it and still impart that sweet flavor. This is particularly true when you use caramelized onion in something that contains liquid, to help the flavor disperse. Just a little caramelized onion in a soup, stew, stir fry or sauce will deliver great flavor.

13. Save pickling brines, broths and vinaigrettes

You'll probably put some effort into making dishes that work safely for P2; some of these creations can multi-task for you.

For example, to be efficient:

— Save the liquid from your **cucumber sunomono salad** (thinly sliced cucumber + rice vinegar + sweetener + salt + fresh mint or ginger, optional) and it later becomes a dressing for cole slaw.

— The **broth you've boiled meatballs in** will taste good later for cooking leafy greens.

— The **"honey mustard" vinaigrette** you made for tuna salad would taste good the next day on cold egg whites or leftover pork tenderloin or as a condiment for a sandwich wrap.

— The **pan juices from when you sautéed mushrooms** will make a good base for whatever your next stir fry is, whether protein or vegetable. Asparagus with prawns would be great cooked in a mushroomy pan. Don't be too proud to stick that sauté pan in the fridge. The leftover umami flavor will be ready for you to use tomorrow.

— The **saffron broth** you made for fresh clams, prawns or fish soup can be used as a stir fry liquid for meat or vegetables.

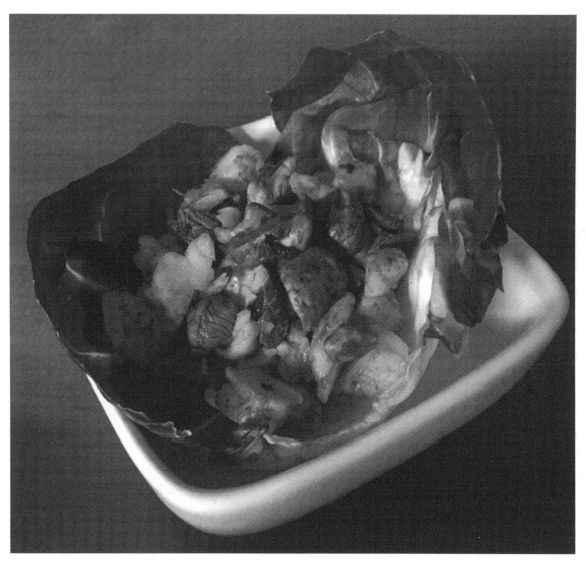

Photo: Dana Falk

The broth leftover from cod and prawn soup was used to sauté diced mushrooms. Leftover prawns from that same soup were chopped and dusted with gumbo seasoning. Together the prawns and mushrooms go into a radicchio cup, which is picked up like a taco.

You can't reuse any liquid that's had raw meat or seafood sitting in it, like a ceviche, but many of the other dressings you make during HCG Phase 2 will multi-task if you give them the chance to. Stock up on tiny storage containers!

14. Meat and veggies minced finely disperse flavor

It may sound obvious, but this trick does help. While a nice, fatty pork shoulder would ooze flavor even if cooked whole, a lean pork tenderloin wouldn't ooze much of anything. Lean meats will disperse their flavor better if they are ground or diced small, rather than left in large pieces. The same holds true for veggies and herbs you are working with.

Some examples:

— You'll get more beef flavor throughout your **beef chili** if you grind the beef than if you cut it into chunks of stew meat.

— Your **mu-shu pork, chicken or shrimp** will be more flavorful if you dice these proteins small rather than using larger pieces.

— You'll create more flavorful **turkey-celery soup**, if you prepare finely chopped turkey and celery, then simmer these in chicken broth longer than you would ordinarily (let's say 60 instead of 30 mins, on low). This will infuse the broth with more flavor than a chunky soup would.

15. Flavorful ingredients may be found in less fancy markets

The cuts of meat that are brutally lean are harder to find at high-end markets, which favor well-marbled cuts. Look for discount grocery stores and supermarkets in more modest neighborhoods. There, you may find **inexpensive cuts of beef like top round**

and round eye. You may find **animal and fish bones for soup**, too, which will add flavor to your P2 cooking, if you have the patience for such things.

At Southeast Asian markets, you may find types of greens that are new to you. There may be types of fish you've never tried that are great for HCG. **Whole fish** are much less expensive per pound than filets are, but they will usually fillet them for free at the seafood counter! That's a good deal if you've got the freezer space.

Herbs tend to be fresher, more diverse and more reasonably priced at ethnic markets, so go looking for **Thai basil and kaffir lime leaves. Halal butchers and Latin markets often have goat meat, mutton** and other HCG-friendly protein options that are more difficult to find at your usual market. Look for vinegars, spices, teas and hot sauces unfamiliar to you, too.

16. If you like spicy food, you're in luck

HCG is a little easier for people who like spicy food. Most of the condiments that bring heat to dishes are perfectly fine on P2. **Soak dried chili peppers in your broth. Add sambal olek or dried red pepper flakes to dishes. Roast hot peppers over an open flame**. Use **wasabi powder or fresh wasabi root**, both of which are hot enough to clear your sinuses and work for P2. If you like things with a little kick but not super spicy, try roasting **mild Anaheim peppers or pasilla peppers**. You can even stuff mild peppers with ground meat and egg whites and bake them in a casserole dish to create **chile relleno**.

Check the label of hot sauces to make sure they doesn't have MSG, sugar or starch. If an ingredient ends in "O-S-E," as in maltodextrose, that's essentially a sugar, metabolically. **Frank's Red Hot** is a good hot sauce choice for HCG. It's worth your while to study labels, since finding just one sauce you love can make a big difference.

17. Roast shellfish in the shell

Prawns, crawfish, lobster and such have lots of flavor in their shells. Rather than peeling and cooking them, **buy prawns and crawfish still in their shell**.

Using **roasted prawns in the shell** as an example: Run a knife along the back of each raw prawn (right through the shell) and scrape out any vein. Toss deveined prawns lightly in salt and roast on a cookie sheet at 400° F. Turn each prawn once, and remove from oven once they are opaque pinkish-orange on both sides. If desired, shake a spice mix on the prawns while still hot. Once cool enough to handle, you've got delicious peel n' eat shrimp.

Not only will the finished shrimp (lobster, crawdads, etc.) be sweeter and deeper in flavor than if you'd peeled them in advance, you'll now have the roasted shells to **make a broth** with. That broth is ideal for simmering veggies in, especially leafy greens. **Bok choy simmered in crab broth?** Yes, please. **Collard greens simmered in crawfish broth?** Completely. **Swiss chard simmered in prawn broth** will taste far better than plain chard does.

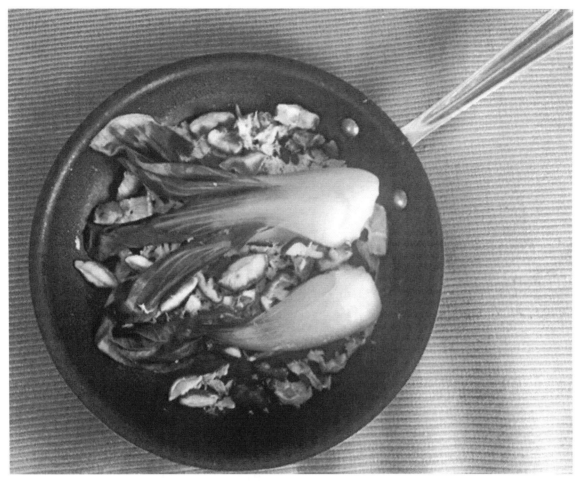

Photo: Dana Falk

Start with enough fat-free chicken broth to cover bottom of skillet. Add leftover crab meat and warm at medium-low. Add shitake mushrooms and baby bok choy (cut in half, face down). Turn heat down to simmer and cook with a lid on until most of the liquid has been absorbed. The result is quite tasty and is super good for HCG.

18. Marinate things you wouldn't ordinarily marinate

One way to impart flavor while on Phase 2 is to consider making a marinade for proteins and veggies you wouldn't normally bother to do this with.

Many of the liquids you'll use on HCG are quite acidic; that's fine for brightening sauces or as a brief marinade, but you don't want food to sit for *too* long in apple cider vinegar or lime juice. If you do, you'll end up with meat that's mushy and fish that's ceviche.

Easy marinade ideas that aren't too acidic:

— Give **ahi tuna** steak some time in a plastic bag with finely chopped **kaffir lime leaves and lemon zest** before grilling it.

— **Turkey breast** that's been sitting in **sage, sherry vinegar and a little sweetener** before it's baked gets a flavor boost.

— Allow your **chicken breasts** to sit in **plain yogurt with tandoori seasoning**; this will tenderize and flavor them, the way it does tandoori chicken. Wipe off the yogurt marinade before baking in a 425° F oven.

— Marinate **pork tenderloin in chai tea**.

— Let your chopped **kale sit in kim chee** before sautéing it, if you like spicy greens.

— Try letting your **asparagus sit in water with lemongrass** before microwaving or stir frying.

— Marinate **shirataki noodles in coconut aminos** to give them a light teriyaki flavor. Drain them well before pan frying.

19. Pounding meat thin helps it take on flavor

This principle always holds true, but it's especially important when on P2. You'll be working with some cuts of meat that need a little help.

To pound your proteins thin, place in a gallon size zipper bag or between two sheets of plastic wrap or parchment paper. If you own a meat pounder, use a light motion and fan outward as you pound the meat, to achieve an even result. If you don't own a meat pounder, you may want to treat yourself to one for this special occasion (you can often find them at thrift stores for a few bucks) or spend about 20 bucks on a nice one, like the *Norpro Grip-EZ Stainless Steel Meat Pounder.* Failing that, wail on your raw turkey breast with a can of kidney beans.

Pound the meat to about 1/4 inch thin. Use the flat of your hand to feel where the meat is not thin enough, then pound lightly to even it out.

If you've used a zipper bag to pound the meat, you'll place this inside of a *second* bag before adding the **marinade, herb pesto, dry rub** or other flavoring, because the outer bag may now have holes. After you've refrigerated the marinated, pounded meat for an hour or so, you'll have a more flavorful finished product.

20. Many herbs and veggies become pesto

Pesto isn't just made with basil and it isn't just for pasta. Traditionally, basil + pine nuts + parmesan cheese + parsley garlic + olive oil + salt = pesto. Several of these ingredients are not shrewd choices for HCG, but happily, you can actually **turn any herbs, spices or soft veggies you wish into a puree that functions like pesto.**

With help from MCT oil as a substitute for olive oil, you can liquify the puree if you need to. Some choices will need this assist to make a smooth puree (as fresh herbs do) and some will not need MCT oil (like most cooked veggies).

Pesto dish ideas:

Fresh spinach + smoked salt pureed with MCT oil = a topping for chicken

Mint + lemongrass + Thai chili pureed = marinade for Mahi Mahi or asparagus

Tarragon + lime zest = topping for ground chicken in lettuce cups

Flat leaf parsley + fresh tomato = topping for egg whites or veal

Spinach + ginger + lemon zest = stuffing for pounded meat that's rolled up

Red bell pepper blanched and pureed + paprika + orange zest = dipping sauce for cold meat leftovers

Arugula + watercress + squeeze lemon juice = peppery sauce for bison meat

Slow cooked tomato + eggplant + fresh thyme = side dish, sauce for white fish, topping for egg whites

21. When you use a slow cooker, 1 + 1 = 3

Using a slow cooker is a great way to coax flavor out of simple ingredients. When you toss a few things in a slow cooker and set it to low heat for 4+ hours, flavors meld and ingredients become tastier than the sum of their parts.

A lean, tough cut of beef like top round cooked with green cabbage, a little well-salted chicken broth and caraway seeds will **mimic corned beef and cabbage** if it spends enough time in a slow cooker. Though you won't have the texture of real corned beef (which is fatty brisket) you will have better tasting beef and better tasting cabbage by allowing them to mingle. That works as social policy and as culinary platform.

More slow cooker ideas:

— **Beef + green bell pepper + Chinese five spice**

— **Chicken + dried shitake mushrooms + fresh ginger**

— **Pork tenderloin + cardamom + rhubarb**

— **Prawns + jalapeño + chayote squash**

— **Lamb sirloin + ras al hanout spice + rosemary + mushrooms**

See if you can come up with other meat, vegetable and spice combinations that would produce the 1 + 1 = 3 effect in your slow cooker.

22. If you like strong coffee, you're in luck

— Coffee tastes better than water does in whey protein isolate shakes, so turn a plain vanilla shake into a **latte shake.**

— Coffee in a **stew or chili** provides depth of flavor.

— Dissolving 1/4 cup unflavored gelatin into 4 cups boiling hot coffee and adding alternative natural sweetener creates **espresso gelatin squares.** It can be a real lifesaver to have a simple dessert like this one utilizing plain coffee. Of course, adding cinnamon or vanilla would make your espresso squares extra special.

— Iced coffee may be more interesting to drink than hot coffee is, especially if you've bought **coffee beans that have a subtle flavor,** like hazelnut (not hazelnut syrup, just hazelnut essence ground coffee). Adding **collagen powder** and blending creates an iced or hot coffee that seems creamy without using cream.

— Finely ground coffee beans may work as a light **crust on steak and meatballs**. If you were to rub down a bison patty with salt, pepper, nutmeg and ground coffee before cooking it in a hot cast iron pan, you'd form a flavorful crust for the burger that goes well with mustard.

If you are not to the type to eat bison burgers rubbed in ground coffee, we understand completely. Reel it in: just try a few new brands of coffee or bring home different roasts within a brand you already like. You may discover both a beverage and an ingredient in the process.

— A touch of coffee in place of water would work as your pan liquid if making **Sloppy Joes.** Sauté ground turkey in a few tablespoons of coffee. Once it's begun to cook, add canned tomatoes, garlic, onion, vinegar and sweetener. Bring the heat to medium low, so the flavor have time to develop. In the finished product, you won't be able to taste coffee, you'll just have a Sloppy Joe that has a little dimension. In the photo that follows, not much canned tomato was added, to save on carbs, but you can create something that looks and tastes more like the Sloppy Joes of your childhood by being more liberal with the crushed tomato component.

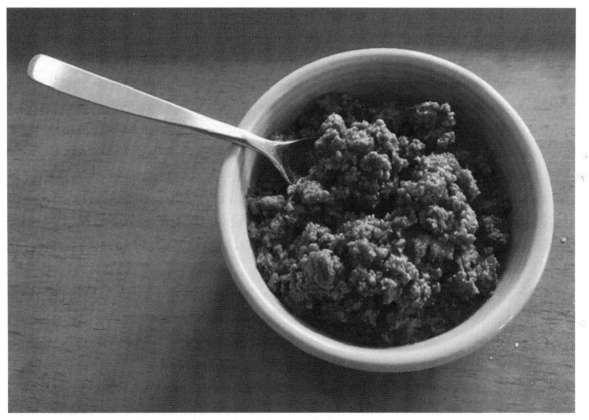

Photo: Dana Falk

Sloppy Joe without the bun isn't beautiful, but it tastes good. Little tricks like sautéing the meat with coffee, to deepen the flavor, help a lot. In a pinch, just lean ground meat + homemade HCG ketchup + salt + dried parsley = Sloppy Joe.

Ideas for Phase 2 Meals

Let's zoom-in now to consider meal prep ideas for HCG Phase 2. Please understand that most of these are recipe *ideas* rather than step-by-step instructions. If you prefer to cook with precise measurements, recipe ideas may be a bit frustrating.

These meal preps are tailored to cooks who like to be given the germ of an idea and run with it (often improving upon the original suggestion). We hope you'll find these meal ideas useful even if that's not your preferred cooking style.

Using ground proteins in HCG cooking

Grinding meat and seafood in your food processor rather than buying it already ground is an important tip for HCG Phase 2. Not only can you better control the fat content, you can incorporate flavor far better than you could by drizzling a sauce on a bland piece of meat or fish. **Meatballs and fish balls cooked in broth** are common in Vietnamese cooking, for example, and it's easy to see why: the protein is gently cooked until tender. The broth is flavored by the cooking protein. It's a win/win, especially for HCG cooking.

You might begin your experimentation with seafood. Some fish, like mahi mahi and, have good flavor and have amazing numbers for HCG. Their protein density scores are 21 and 23 respectively, which is spectacular. If you make croquettes by putting either of these fish through a food processor and adding complementary flavors, you've got something you can eat a huge portion of. You could make **mahi mahi or snapper croquettes** by processing them with fairly delicate flavors like lemongrass, chervil, celeriac (celery root), cilantro or fennel. Maybe a little curry powder or fenugreek. Maybe a dash of fish sauce or tamari. Keep it simple and you'll have little croquettes you can eat in a lettuce wrap. You can bake your croquettes or simmer them in broth. Cook them gently, so they won't get rubbery.

As for animal proteins, there's a reason meatloaf is usually a mixture of ground veal, beef and pork: the flavor and texture are improved upon by the combination. You can of course make all-turkey, veal or bison meatballs if you prefer those excellent protein density scores.

How do you make meatballs tender when you can't use bread crumbs? A little raw egg white, a fresh mushroom or two pulverized, a pinch of unflavored gelatin powder — all of these work. They all work together, too. This technique has nothing much to do with flavor; it's a way to make the *texture* of any ground meat filling more tender. Adding any of these ingredients would improve the texture of your meat filling for **stuffed peppers, stuffed cabbage rolls and chile relleno**, too.

Keeping some fully cooked, **homemade meatballs** in the freezer will save your tail on more than one occasion. It's a quick snack, dipped in "honey mustard." A leftover meatball may be crumbled in your morning egg whites. It may be wrapped with kim chee in a sheet of nori.

Meatballs may easily be served to friends as an appetizer with a sauce you can eat but they will also enjoy. If you prefer, offer two sauces: one you can eat on HCG and one store-bought sauce that they will appreciate.

TIP: We're thinking of "meatballs" here as any little nuggets you have made by adding flavor to ground meat or fish. These could be **kofta, kibbedeh, fish croquettes, prawn dumplings** and such, not just classic meatballs.

For P2 cooking, meatballs may be baked on a cookie sheet, popped in a toaster oven or sautéed in a well-seasoned cast iron pan without oil. All of these will provide a little browning, though none will give you the crust that pan frying fatty meat would, of course.

If you form your ground, spiced meat around a single skewer and flatten it slightly, you've got **kofta.** Kofta is made in North Africa, the Middle East and some parts of the Mediterranean. Cook your ground meat skewer on an outdoor grill if you have that opportunity; there's no flavor better than that. Kofta don't actually have to be one long piece and they don't have to be on a skewer. Many people form them into the shape of small, flattened footballs and cook them in a cast iron pan. Either way, the strategy is this: use your hands to get herbs and spices into ground meat, then grill it.

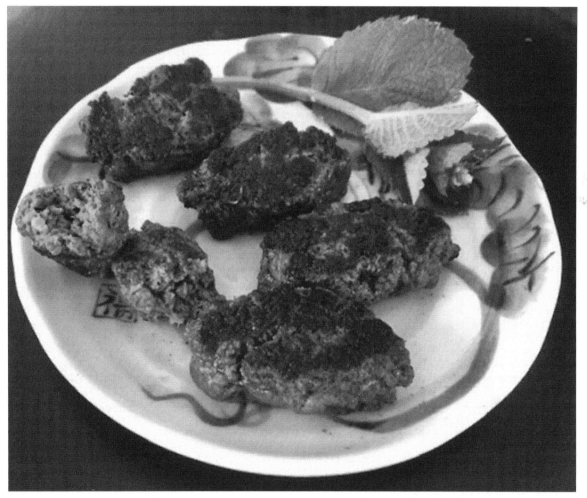

Photo: Dana Falk

Kofta made with lamb sirloin, mint, garlic, a little onion, smoked salt and cinnamon. These were browned in a seasoned, cast iron pan — with no oil! Kofta may also be grilled on a skewer.

The herbs and spices in kofta recipes generally look like this:

Lots of fresh chopped cilantro, mint or flat leaf parsley
Garlic
Salt and pepper
Sumac or paprika (or both)
Cinnamon (highly recommended)
Cumin and coriander
Optional: cayenne powder or chili paste

Whether you make meatballs or kofta, they will taste mighty fine eaten cold the next day. Toss in a zipper bag and eat with your fingers while stuck in traffic.

If you make a batch of meatballs or kofta all the same weight (let's say each meatball 20 grams) you'll know how much you've eaten just by counting the meatballs. Your meal will then be super easy to enter on the tracking app of your choice. We depart from the original Simeons HCG protocol in that we do not believe that all of your protein servings must be exactly 100 grams, but it's still nice to have your dishes portioned.

Flavor profiles for meatballs

A few of the flavor ideas below have a preferred cooking method associated with them. For example, the gyro croquettes, the kofta and the kibbeh might be best cooked in a cast iron pan or on a grill, to get some crust. The Thai fish balls might ideally be gently simmered in soup. In general though, your experimentation is key. If you create just one kind of meatball you love that works for Phase 2, you'll be in good shape.

Consider trying these flavor profiles:

— **Vietnamese meatballs** with chicken, lemongrass, hot chiles and fish sauce.

— **Eastern European meatballs** with pork tenderloin, cabbage and smoked paprika.

— **Moroccan kofta** with ground lamb, cinnamon, fresh mint and lemon zest.

— **Middle Eastern gyro croquettes** with beef, lamb or chicken in any combination and shwarma seasoning mix.

— **Cajun seafood croquettes** with pureed raw crawfish, prawns, catfish or tilapia. Add finely diced bell pepper and a tiny bit of onion you've sautéed with gumbo file spice mix in chicken broth. Form into small patties and bake on both sides.

— **Persian kibbeh** with beef and allspice, cumin, curry powder and a small amount of grated onion. (Traditional kibbeh has bulgur wheat, which doesn't work for P2, but add a little cauliflower rice for texture, if you wish.)

— **Thai fish balls** (*Tod Mun Pla*) with your choice of white fish, like red snapper, orange roughy or cod. Use raw prawns if you prefer a firmer texture. Puree the raw seafood then add a little fish sauce, mild curry powder and chopped coriander leaves (cilantro). Sprinkle a bit of konjac root powder if you have it, to help bind, or incorporate some egg white.

Refrigerate the mixture before forming into balls or patties. *Tod Mun Pla* fish balls are typically deep fried, but baking them or simmering in soup works too.

— **Chinese meatballs** with ground beef or bison. Grind the meat in your food processor an extra long time, until very smooth. Add pureed fresh ginger, ground shitake mushrooms, Chinese five spice and a little tamari or coconut aminos.

If you want to mimic those delicious **steamed dim sum meatballs,** add to your beef mixture 1 tsp unflavored gelatin you have bloomed in 3 tbs of boiling water. Add a little chopped cilantro or flat leaf parsley and steam the meatballs until cooked through. If you don't want them dim sum style, leave out the gelatin and bake your meatballs at 350 degrees and keep an eye on them so they won't dry out.

— **Italian style meatballs** may be made for P2 with any meat you like. Game meats like venison or elk, pork tenderloin, lean beef, bison or ground turkey will all work; turkey breast and game meat will have the best protein density scores.

Add good salt, pepper if you like it, chopped flat leaf parsley, pureed garlic, fresh or dried oregano and a little tomato you have charred on the stove. (Go light on the oregano unless you adore it; it's a potent flavor that can hijack a dish.) Sauté your meatballs in a well-seasoned cast iron pan or bake on a cookie sheet.

Meat Beyond Meatballs

Classic Meatloaf

Think about meatloaf's first cousins: **stuffed bell peppers, Russian cabbage rolls, chile relleno, baked zucchini boats, stuffed mushrooms.** Anything you can stuff with meat you can stuff with meatloaf, which will be far more tasty. Your own special ground meat blend is key to a variety of dishes for HCG.

It's common to put ketchup in classic meatloaf. If you want to do this while on HCG, be sure you work with your own homemade HCG ketchup made of crushed or strained tomatoes, not with traditional ketchup or tomato paste. Tomato paste has concentrated sugars. Traditional ketchup has corn syrup or sugar.

Pomi Brand tomato products, which come in a box rather than a can, are high quality and tend to be relatively low in carbs. Adding apple cider vinegar and an alternative natural sweetener would produce your own **HCG-friendly ketchup.** Increasingly, there are sugar free ketchups on the market, too, some of which would work for HCG.

Hot and Sour Soup with Meatballs

Your hot and sour meatball **soup base** will be fat free chicken broth or stock, unless you've made some stock of your own. To get it "hot," use fresh grated ginger or galanga and dry Thai chili flakes or red pepper flakes. To get it "sour," use fresh lime juice and minced lemongrass. To give it more depth (optional) add a dash of fish sauce and a dash of coconut aminos. Taste your soup base for the balance of hot and sour that you enjoy and adjust as needed. Once you find the right balance, your hot and sour soup broth will be liquid gold for a round of HCG. After you've eaten it as soup, your hot and sour broth doubles as cooking liquid for another dish. Hot and sour soup is very versatile so make a big batch.

To make **hot and sour soup with meatballs**, add shirataki noodles and sliced mushrooms to bulk out your broth. Finally, add the raw meatballs and let simmer in the hot soup at medium low until they're cooked through. The finished meatballs can then simmer gently on very lowest heat for quite a while and as they do, they will taste more and more like your hot and sour broth.

More Meaty Ideas

If you want look up a classic recipe for any of these dishes and cannot find ones tailored to the HCG Diet, make those adjustments yourself. You know how to choose lean proteins, how to choose low carb veggies, how to cook with broth instead of oil and which fresh herbs and dried spices are your favorites.

More ideas for meat dishes:

Top round beef stew with turnips

Chicken adobo in the slow cooker

Curried goat with okra

Buffalo spice chicken breast

Venison and mushroom kabobs

Cinnamon anise pork in the slow cooker

Turkey salad in half a bell pepper

Button mushrooms stuffed with veal and parsley

Pork tenderloin with sauerkraut and "honey mustard"

The Twelve Most Versatile Vegetables

Veggies will be a pretty big part of your daily life when on HCG. If you choose the right vegetables, they're something you can eat in large amounts on the diet. Some vegetables are particularly good staples to keep in the house, because there are so many ways to put them to work.

1. Asparagus

One of the many things asparagus has going for it is how serving hot and cold both work. This is not true of all vegetables, to be sure. The recipe for microwave asparagus [below] works well as a cold salad the following day, for example.

Another virtue is the texture options you have when cooking asparagus: thin asparagus spears prepared *al dente* (slightly crisp) is a different beast from thick asparagus, cooked until soft. Because the HCG stats for asparagus are so fantastic — it's a Tier 1 veggie, so you can eat a whole lot of it — it's to your advantage to find at least one preparation of it you enjoy.

Third, **asparagus plays well with a wide variety of flavors.** Fresh herbs, like mint, are a natural. Dried herbs, like Herbs de Provence, are a French classic. Using citrus juice and zest gives you a light, fresh taste. (Grapefruit is especially awesome with asparagus.) Sesame seeds, fresh ginger and a dash of tamari produce an Asian flavor.

DANA FALK, PH.D. & KELSEY KLAUSMEYER, N.D.

Asparagus that's been simply cooked in a microwave is surprisingly tasty, considering how spartan it is. This side dish makes a handy, complete dinner when you end up with very few calories left for the day.

Microwave Asparagus

— Break off the woody ends of 1 pound of asparagus.
— Use a fork to poke multiple holes in each spear.
— Toss in 2 tsp good quality salt. (This is more salt than you would ordinarily use.)
— Add 1/4 tsp fresh, grated nutmeg.

Optional additions: crushed celery seeds, red pepper flakes.

— Let the salted asparagus sit raw for 20 minutes.
— Place in a shallow pan that will fit in your microwave. Add enough water to barely cover the bottom of the dish.
— Microwave on high for 2-3 minutes.

For those who like crisp asparagus, it may be done at this point.

For those who like it more tender, toss the asparagus in the salty water and return to microwave until it reaches your preferred doneness.

Optional but really delicious:
Finish with a squeeze of grapefruit and some fresh mint or fresh basil.

Chop up your leftover microwave asparagus to make a **cold asparagus and prawn salad** the next day.

When asparagus is boiled until soft, then pureed with vegetable broth or chicken broth to your desired consistency, you have the base of **cream of asparagus soup.** Now add to taste: sea salt, grated nutmeg, fresh tarragon, a dash of sherry vinegar if you've got it.

In spring and summer you may find fresh **white asparagus** at the market, which is incredibly tender, and purple asparagus, which would make a fun side dish. Fresh white asparagus is much milder in flavor than green asparagus is (less grassy, more floral) and it is more delicate in texture (not stringy the way green asparagus can be). It's in season late spring, usually. It's not cheap, but you might consider buying **white asparagus in a jar or tin** when it's not in season. Check the label, but you'll generally find that it's fine from a jar for HCG.

Treating yourself to a jar or tin of gourmet white asparagus is a good example of splurging on a gourmet food for this special occasion. While you're on P2, finding something delicious to eat is vital to your stamina for the diet, so grab those foods when you find them.

2. Red and Orange Bell Peppers

Many people miss tasting sweetness when on HCG, especially if they're choosing not to use alternative natural sweeteners. Utilizing the natural sweetness of red and orange bell peppers is a nice help. They're crisp and somewhat sweet when raw; tender and have balanced sweetness when cooked. Yellow and green bell peppers are an option as well — in fact they have fewer carbs than the red and orange peppers do — but we'll focus here on how to utilize the sweetness of red and orange peppers.

Baking stuffed bell peppers is genius on P2. It's one of those foods that doesn't look like you're on a special diet. The meat or veg filling you make is adapted to your preferred flavors: you can make filling spicy or garlicky, full of fresh herbs or all veggie. Stuffed bell peppers freeze well (after baking) and have really good numbers for HCG Phase 2.

Such a compelling argument for a batch of stuffed bell peppers! Here's how you'd make six servings.

Stuffed Bell Peppers
Six servings

3 large red or orange bell peppers
1 egg white
1 pound raw HCG meat of choice, ground
1.5 tbs HCG friendly ketchup
1.5 tbs grated or minced onion
1 clove garlic, grated on microplane or minced
1/8 tsp grated nutmeg
3/4 tsp kosher salt

Optional:
Dried shitake mushrooms, pulverized
Cauliflower rice
Diced jalapeños
Fresh basil, tarragon, oregano or parsley
Red pepper flakes

— Preheat oven to 400 degrees.

— Line a cookie sheet with parchment paper or foil or give a pyrex glass pan a very light spray of oil.

— Cut three large red or orange bell peppers in half lengthwise. These six halves will be your six servings. Remove seeds and papery pith.

— Make sure your pound of raw, ground meat is fully thawed. Season raw meat with salt, nutmeg, garlic and onion.

— Whip an egg white by hand until frothy. Add to the seasoned raw meat.

— Add the HCG ketchup.

— Add any of the optional ingredients you're using, like fresh herbs, spices or cauliflower rice. Cauliflower rice gives you some of the texture that's normally in stuffed peppers; it bulks out your filling, so you may have some meat leftover for meatballs.

— Divide the meat filling among the six pepper halves.

— Bake the peppers 35 minutes at 375° F degrees, then start testing for doneness. Internal temperature of the meat should be at least 160° F.

— After 35 mins, turn the oven up to 400° F and bake for the final 10 mins.

If you'd like more char on the peppers than what you see in the photo, increase the oven to 425° F and keep an eye on them. The cooking time will vary depending upon how large the cavity of the peppers is and how thickly stuffed they are.

— Enjoy! Leftovers freeze well if wrapped individually.

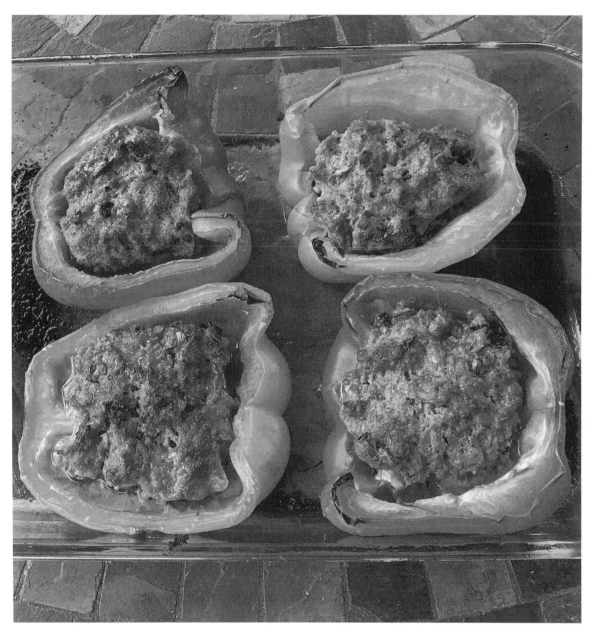

Photo: Dana Falk

Stuffed peppers made with ground turkey, dried shitake mushrooms and fresh basil. Give them a blast of 450° F heat for the last five minutes in the oven if you want more char around the edges.

In general, bell peppers love high heat and high heat loves them back. If you have a gas stove you can **char whole peppers over an open flame.** If you don't, you can put whole or half peppers on a cookie sheet in a 450° F oven, then finish them under the broiler.

Bell peppers are a natural for an outdoor grill. If you barbecue shish-kebab, alternating chunks of red or orange bell pepper with button mushrooms and a protein, you'll have a colorful, flavorful meal. If you can afford the carbs, add a single layer of onion between each mushroom and pepper.

Raw, whole bell peppers are sturdy: they can take a little abuse bouncing around in your backpack or car while maintaining integrity and crunch. If you bring sliced red pepper along as a snack — and that may frankly be its strongest suit while on HCG — you can create some sweet and sour crunch. Try **squeezing lime juice and sprinkling a little sea salt** on pieces of red bell pepper. That sounds pitiful, doesn't it? But you'd be surprised how something crunchy, salty, sweet and sour hits the spot when you're really hungry.

A whole, raw pepper cut in half with seeds and white pith removed also makes a sturdy **vessel for tuna or chicken salad.** Same goes for leftover **blackened crawfish or plain crab meat** as a filling. Thinly julienned raw red or orange bell pepper may also add color and flavor to your green cabbage **cole slaw.**

Talk about versatile — bell pepper can also be transformed into a **savory red bell pepper sauce** that's slightly sweet. It's good as a sauce for dry meat like chicken or turkey breast, it adds some interest to plain egg whites, dresses up steamed veggies like broccoli with flavor and color. Better yet, red bell pepper sauce can be your substitute for mayonnaise when you make a sandwich wrap out of luncheon meat or nori sheets.

Red Bell Pepper Sauce

This sauce is usually thickened with soaked cashews, olive oil or shallot puree; all things you cannot use right now. The HCG version will be too thin if you leave out the eggplant.

2 large red bell peppers, cubed
1/2 - 3/4 cup eggplant, cubed
1/2 garlic clove
1/2 Serrano or jalapeño pepper (or more, to taste)
Up to 3/4 cup chicken or mushroom broth

1/4 small onion (less if it's a large onion)
or 1/4 small green apple (or a blend of the two)

1 tbs lemon juice
1 - 2 dashes red or white wine vinegar
1/8 - 1/4 tsp sweet (mild) paprika
Optional: Fistful of fresh basil leaves

Optional, but yummy: Allspice, saffron, fenugreek, smoked pepper, nutmeg

— Bake the peppers, eggplant and 1/4 onion or apple on a cookie sheet at 400° F for 15-17 mins. Once softened, remove from oven.
— Puree hot veggies in a food processor.
— Add 1/2 of the broth, puree again.
— Add remaining ingredients except for broth, puree.
— Add remaining broth 1 tsp at a time, until sauce is to desired thickness.

3. Collard greens

Collards have large, sturdy leaves. Of course you can make traditional **Southern collard greens** by removing the center vein and ripping them into pieces. You then simmer them in broth and bones, cider vinegar, onions and garlic, a little smoked paprika and hot sauce. This works for mustard greens and turnip greens, too, though these don't need to simmer for as long as collards do.

You can also use the sturdiness of the leaves to create a **collard sandwich wrap.** Soften a single whole collard leaf by boiling it or microwaving with salted water in a shallow dish until very pliable. Once cool, roll in your sandwich filling (let's say rotisserie chicken, tomato and jalapeño mustard). The collard leaf should be strong enough to work as a wrap.

4. Celery

The anchor of the dull vegetable tray is under-appreciated. We recommend you buy the whole celery, leaves included, not just the cleaned, trimmed celery ribs.

Celery is delicious when **roasted in the oven or braised in flavorful garlic broth.** Celery bulks out your tuna or chicken salad. Keep some in the refrigerator in salted water. It will be extra crisp with extra flavor when you reach for it.

If you decide to eat a little dairy while on HCG (for example, some non-fat cottage cheese) you can make celery a more filling snack by creating **herbed cheese spread** to put inside it. Drain the cottage cheese very well in a mesh strainer. If time allows, putting it on top of a paper towel *inside* that strainer and leaving it overnight will make your finished product extra dense and satisfying.

Place your drained cottage cheese in a bowl. Using a hand mixer, blend in any combination of fresh thyme, tarragon, mint, dill, basil or chervil. Use any of your favorite herbs, as long as they are *fresh*, not dried. Add lemon, lime or orange zest, a small squeeze of citrus juice, a medium pinch of salt and (optional) a pinch of fenugreek, lemongrass or curry powder. Cream with a hand mixer and you'll have an herbed cheese spread to fill ribs of celery. If you want to bulk out the herbed cheese spread, finely mince some bell pepper and incorporate. You might serve herbed cheese spread on crackers to company, while yours would be served inside celery, mini bell peppers or **Belgian endive.**

Celery *leaves* are also under-appreciated; they taste light and fresh and are slightly bitter. The leaves are good in a **soup base, on top of cold noodle bowls, in chicken salad and are great on top of cold, hard boiled eggs.** Celery leaves will not form the base of a meal, but they're a lovely and fresh-tasting garnish.

5. Radishes

Radishes are fantastic for HCG. You can eat radishes cut in half with salt and lime juice. You can make salads crunchier. You can **pickle radishes or buy radish kim chee.** Farmer's Markets often have colorful **purple, pink or white heirloom varieties** that are less peppery in flavor than the red radishes we're accustomed to. Latino markets sometimes sell large bags of red radishes that have already been cleaned and trimmed and are reasonably priced. Korean markets often have a large selection of radish varieties. Look carefully at the options: some radishes are large, some are small and some don't look like what you might think of as a radish.

Not only do radishes provide crunch, they can do the opposite! **When over-cooked, radishes can ice used to imitate potatoes.** You know that dim sum called "pan-fried turnip cake?" That is cooked, mashed radish (with rice flour added to make it hold together and crisp up). All radishes become milder when over-cooked. To make radish mashers, peel the mildest radishes you can find. Dice, then boil with a garlic clove thrown into the boiling water. Cook until tender, drain the water and garlic, then mash the softened radishes or put them through a potato ricer.

Perhaps you'd prefer to keep your **boiled or steamed radishes in cube form** and use them in recipes to emulate potatoes: in slow cooker meats, in curries, in soups. Bulk out the filling of your cabbage rolls for very few calories with cooked, cubed radish. All alone, boiled radish is not a treat — but it's a clever hack for HCG Phase 2.

6. Cauliflower

Cauliflower is remarkably useful because you can really play with the form it takes. Plain cauliflower rice comes in bags, or you may chop it finely yourself in your food processor. This gives the cauliflower the texture of couscous or rice, so it works as a side dish for your protein. Simmer your **cauliflower rice** in a small amount of broth, with curry powder or saffron and a little nutmeg, to impart some flavor and color. If you've already made roasted garlic paste, cauliflower rice would be a great use for it; just a dab of that concentrated flavor would give you garlic cauliflower rice.

Whole heads of cauliflower may be sliced thick to create a **cauliflower steak.** Slice a head of cauliflower into one-inch thick slices. Steam or microwave for 90 minutes to soften a bit, then grill it like a steak. You cannot use MCT Oil to coat your pan, but you can create a spice rub for your cauliflower, then grill in a well-seasoned cast iron pan. **Indian flavors** work well for cauliflower steaks, so consider garam masala, coriander, curry powder and cardamom in your rub. **Smoky flavors** work well too, so consider a rub of cherrywood smoked salt and smoked paprika.

Roasted cauliflower salad is another of those HCG dishes that you could serve to friends and they'd have no idea you're on a special diet.

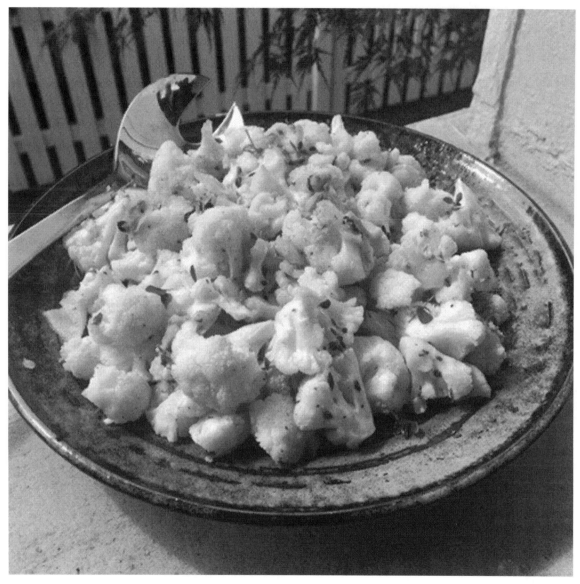

Photo: Dana Falk

Roasted cauliflower salad here was made with lemon vinaigrette, allspice and lemon thyme. It's filling, has good flavor, lasts a while in the fridge and travels well to potlucks and picnics.

Roasted Cauliflower Salad

Salad
1 head of cauliflower
1/4 medium green apple, peeled
1/2 tsp kosher salt
1/8 tsp pepper
1/8 tsp ground allspice and/or nutmeg (more if you love it)
1 clove garlic, grated
4 tsp (total) fresh chopped herbs of choice: fennel fronds, thyme, dill, tarragon, basil, flat leaf parsley or cilantro. (Fennel fronds and thyme would both taste awesome.)

Dressing
1 tbs MCT oil
2 tbs lemon juice
1 tsp Swerve confectioners or equivalent sweetener
Pinch salt
1/2 of the fresh herbs (2 tsp)

This does not make a lot of dressing; it's enough to lightly coat the cauliflower and give it a pleasing lemon flavor. If you want a more moist salad, like a pasta salad, make more vinaigrette.

— Preheat oven to 375° F degrees.

— Cut cauliflower into small florets, discard stem.

— Roughly chop fresh herb(s) of choice.

— Place a mat, parchment or foil on a cookie sheet. Add cauliflower florets and 1/2 of the fresh herbs (2 teaspoons).

— Use the largest section of your grater and roughly grate the apple directly onto cauliflower and herbs. If you don't have a large grater, slice the apple as thinly as possible, then chop it.

— Toss all in salt, pepper, allspice and/or nutmeg.

— Bake at 375° F degrees for 20 minutes, rotating pan and tossing cauliflower at the 10 minute mark.

— Remove pan and let cool a few minutes.

The cauliflower will be just slightly browned when you remove it and it will not be soft. This prevents the garlic from burning and keeps the finished salad slightly crunchy.

— While the cauliflower is cooling, make the dressing. Whisk MCT oil, lemon juice and sweetener thoroughly. Incorporate salt and fresh herbs.

— Toss warm cauliflower mixture with lemon vinaigrette dressing.

— Serve chilled or at room temperature. Tastes best if has been in dressing for several hours before serving.

If instead you want **cauliflower hummus,** roast cauliflower florets well, then puree with a little chopped raw garlic, lemon juice, MCT oil and fresh parsley. If you want more authentic middle eastern flavor, sprinkle with sumac. This hummus would be especially nice served in endive leaves or mini sweet bell peppers.

For a **cauliflower mash**, boil florets with a clove of garlic in heavily salted water or broth. Drain *very* well, then puree in a food processor with nutmeg. Without butter, you probably won't mistake cauliflower mash for mashed potatoes, but it's a nice side dish for HCG. If you want to make the taste more complex, add some **cooked celeriac** (also called celery root) along with the raw cauliflower to the boiling liquid. Celeriac (Tier 4) is higher carb than cauliflower (Tier 2) is, but even 1/4 cup of celeriac will add gorgeous flavor.

You know that fancy **yellowish-orange cauliflower** you never buy because it's more expensive than the white cauliflower? The yellow-orange varieties are a bit sweeter in flavor and creamier in texture than white cauliflower is and they have the same number of carbs. (Some sources list the fancy varieties as having fewer carbs, actually.) Perhaps you'll treat yourself to the heirloom varieties of cauliflower while on HCG. The orange cauliflower would make a beautiful puree as a side dish or the base of a cream of cauliflower soup.

Cream of cauliflower soup is a delightful freak of nature, since it tastes creamy without using any cream. If you're in a big hurry, you could make a **quick n' dirty cauliflower soup** by cooking a bag of cauliflower rice in broth until soft. Drain well and puree. Then add the broth a little at a time to achieve the consistency you like. Finish with a good amount of salt, pepper and nutmeg.

If you want a **gourmet cream of cauliflower soup**, make your cauliflower puree out of two styles of cauliflower: half will be florets you've browned in the oven with salt and half will be plain boiled cauliflower you've pureed. Puree these two together, drizzling chicken broth to thin it to your desired soup consistency. Optional: add a splash of sherry vinegar or apple cider vinegar. Finish with fresh thyme.

7. Cabbage

Turn cabbage into **mu-shu chicken** by slicing it thinly and stir-frying it with chicken and mushrooms. Nice additions, if you have them, are bamboo shoots (3.6 carbs) and shirataki noodles. Your sauté sauce will be coconut aminos, a dash of rice vinegar, a dash of fish sauce (optional) and a pinch of Chinese five spice. Add grated fresh ginger for more intense flavor.

Real mu-shu has some scrambled egg in the dish. You can do that if you don't mind using your one, precious whole egg in this way. We suggest you taste the stir fry first to see if it's tasty enough already that you don't need the egg.

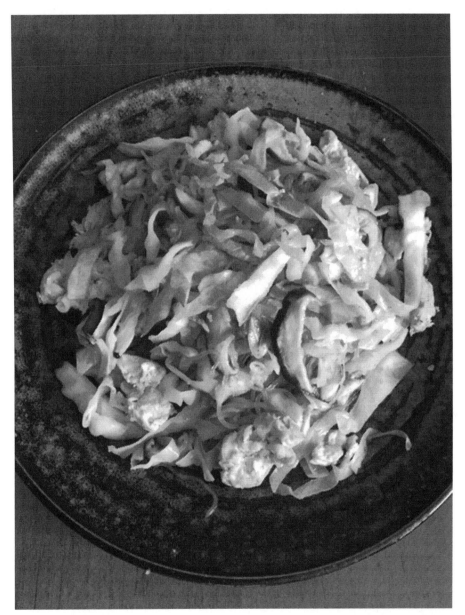

Photo: Dana Falk

Mu-shu chicken made with shitake mushrooms and angel hair shirataki noodles. The noodles were marinated in coconut aminos and cooked in a dry pan before other ingredients were added.

To make **cabbage rolls**, boil or steam whole cabbage leaves to make them pliable. Fill with ground meat of choice and bulk out that filling with grated zucchini, cooked spinach, chopped sautéed mushrooms, cooked radishes or cauliflower rice — essentially any P2 veggie that you can use a lot of.

Next, make a batch of **sweet and sour tomato sauce**: Pomi crushed tomato + apple cider vinegar + salt + chopped flat parsley or chopped fresh basil + sweetener + grated nutmeg (optional). Spread a small amount of sauce in the bottom of a glass pan. Place your cabbage rolls in the baking pan and cover with more sauce.

Bake cabbage rolls at 350 degrees until meat inside is 160° F, about 40 minutes. Baking time will depend upon how much meat you've put in each roll, of course. You may wish to make just a few large cabbage rolls that you intend to eat as one meal apiece, which makes tracking the nutrition easy.

Cabbage is also versatile because you can purchase it already shredded in a bag. Use shredded cabbage for mu-shu or cole slaw. A super quick **cole slaw dressing** would be a little non-fat yogurt you have diluted with your vinegar of choice and alternative natural sweetener of choice.

You can throw some cabbage in a slow cooker or dutch oven with whatever meat you're making and it will take on the flavor of the meat. Try **veal with cabbage in the slow cooker**; veal has a mild flavor and is more tender than the other lean meats on Phase 2. The result will be a bit like corned beef and cabbage.

Shabu-shabu is thinly sliced, raw meat or seafood with vegetables that you cook at the table, in a bowl of bubbling hot broth. Napa cabbage and enoki mushrooms are common components of shabu-shabu, but shitake mushrooms are lower in carbs than enoki are, so consider the substitution. It's a healthy, fun meal to share with others. Yours won't be eaten over the traditional sticky rice, but you can use cauliflower rice or shirataki noodles if you wish in place of rice. In essence, it's cook-at-the-table cabbage soup that's fun to share.

Try using the more tender varieties of cabbage, like **savoy and napa cabbages as a cup for Thai larb.** These varieties are less dense than the tightly packed heads of green cabbage. Some people are not crazy about the cruciferous flavor of green cabbage; they prefer the less assertive flavor of napa and savoy cabbages.

Cabbage is very filling and has awesome specs for HCG; see if you can work it into your rotation, even just as a jar of kim chee or sauerkraut.

8. Radicchio

Radicchio is beautiful to look at, with its purple leaves and white veins and it's very useful for P2. Radicchio is more tender than cabbage is and the shape of its leaves form a natural cup. This means it's a natural for holding leftover meat, like Thai larb with lime juice or a chicken salad with MCT vinaigrette.

Radicchio adds color to an ordinary salad or cole slaw when thinly sliced; even if you don't love its slightly bitter flavor, it serves a purpose.

A head of radicchio is sturdy, with tightly packed leaves — intelligent design for holding together nicely if you want to cut it in half and make **grilled radicchio**. Salt it, grill in a cast iron pan for maximum char, then drizzle with sherry vinegar, tarragon vinegar or MCT lemon vinaigrette while still warm. Extra points for spotting the *When Harry Met Sally* reference.

Finally, radicchio is considered somewhat fancy — it's not cheap — so perhaps you would serve it to company if you need to entertain while you're on Phase 2. Serving **ground**

larb, shrimp salad, egg salad, ahi poke, crawfish or ceviche in a radicchio cup would not even tip people off that you're eating carefully.

9. Cucumbers

Cucumbers punch above their weight. They may be **pickled** and eaten as a side dish. See separate section, called "Veggies You Could Pickle." Those pickles, made without sugar, may be chopped to make a relish. Add a little alternative natural sweetener for a sweet relish to add to tuna.

Cucumbers give any **sandwich wrap** more crunch. Cucumbers may be put through a spiralizer to create a pretty, **twirly salad.** They may be sliced thin and left in a pitcher of water to make **cucumber-infused water,** which you could drink chilled or use to make an amazing cup of tea. Cucumbers may be or **hollowed out and filled with tuna.** They're inexpensive, low calorie, sturdy enough for travel and very filling. Small **Persian cucumbers** and crunchy **pickling cucumbers** are especially sturdy for travel.

Greek Salad is a great use of cucumbers: Diced cucumber + diced tomato + small amount dried oregano + lemon juice + salt, pepper.

English cucumbers are great for making a side dish called **Sichuan smashed cucumber salad** (*pai huang gua*). English cucumbers are long, with a thin skin and vertical ridges; they often come individually wrapped in plastic.

Sichuan smashed cucumber salad (*pai huang gua*)

— Trim the ends from two English cucumbers, leaving the peel on.

— Cut each cucumber into 3-4 pieces.

— Place inside a large zipper bag and bash the cucumbers with a meat tenderizer, flat side of a cleaver, heavy pan or heavy bottle of oil. (You know you've resorted to it before.) Don't beat the cucumbers to a pulp, just give them a whack, breaking them down.

— Place the smashed English cucumbers in a colander over a bowl or the sink and allow liquid to drain. Toss 1.5 - 2 teaspoons kosher salt into the cucumbers and let sit in the colander for 30 minutes. You'll see that several tablespoons of liquid drain in that half hour! This makes the cucumbers extra crisp and a little briny.

— While the cucumbers are draining, make the **dressing**:

1/4 cup coconut aminos
1 tbs rice vinegar or black vinegar
Zest and juice of 1 small lime
1 tbs MCT oil
1 1/2 tsp fish sauce
1 1/2 tsp grated garlic
1 tsp grated ginger

Optional:
4 drops stevia glycerite or equivalent alternative natural sweetener
1/2 tsp (or more) minced Thai chiles
Grated fresh jalapeño
Red pepper flakes or hot sauce

— Whisk dressing ingredients together and adjust to taste. Set aside.

The longer the dressing sits before you use it as a marinade, the more the ginger and garlic will reward you with gorgeous flavor.

— After the smashed cucumbers have drained in the colander, use your fingers to break the smashed cucumbers into smaller, bite-sized pieces. They will be very irregular.

— Transfer to a mixing bowl and toss with your dressing. Let marinate at least 15 minutes before eating; ideally one hour.

— After the cucumber has marinated in the dressing for an hour, drain it and save the dressing for some other dish.

Your *pai huang gua* may be served chilled or at room temperature.

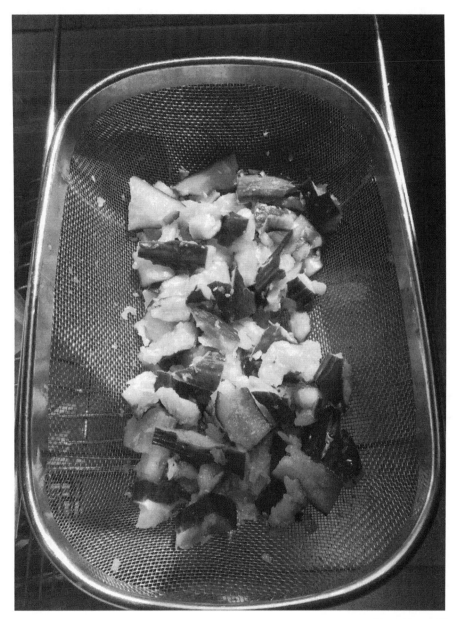

Photo: Dana Falk

After English cucumbers get a cathartic smack in a plastic bag, the pieces will look irregular. The kosher salt you sprinkle on makes liquid drain through the colander, producing crisp and briny cucumber bits.

Sichuan smashed cucumber salad would make a nice fresh **side dish for a lemongrass pork, a spicy chicken stir fry or a lemon baked fish.**

Traditionally, *pai huang gua* is eaten with a drizzle of sesame oil, a drizzle of chili oil and some toasted sesame seeds. These three ingredients don't work for HCG, but if you like this dish enough to keep it in your repertoire, you'll like it even better in a few months, when you can finish it with more flavor.

10. Mushrooms

Mushrooms make everything they touch taste earthier, more savory, more interesting. They may also be used to add moisture to a recipe, like meatloaf, because they put off liquid when they cook.

Mushrooms are an example of a vegetable that varies a lot in carbohydrate by the *variety* you select, so do your homework before grocery shopping. Tiny enoki mushrooms have 8 grams carbs per 100 grams (Tier 4) but enormous, meaty portobello mushrooms have only 3.5 carbs (Tier 1.) You could put a **marinated portobello mushroom on the grill** and eat the whole thing; it's the size of a burger! Serve with buns to others, eat your own as a lettuce wrap.

You can also make **stuffed portobello mushrooms** by baking rather than grilling. Your stuffing may be a combination of ground meat and veggies, for example veal, spinach and egg white with garlic. Because they give off liquid while baking, placing portobellos on a rack inside a baking sheet will produce the best results.

Shitake mushrooms are delicious and offer the added benefit of being chewy, which is a mouth feel you don't get much of while on HCG. Fresh prawn, asparagus and shitake mushroom stir fry could seriously be served at a dinner party. It won't taste the same as it would stir-fried with peanut oil, but it'll taste pretty darn good. Try sautéing the prawn-asparagus-shitake dish in **ginger-infused chicken broth.** Be sure to trim the stems of shitake mushrooms; they are woody and do not soften much during cooking.

Fresh shitake mushrooms are fairly expensive. What are surprisingly affordable are ***dried shitake mushrooms***. Dried shitakes you've **pulverized into a powder** in your coffee bean grinder make meatloaf taste good without the breadcrumbs. That powder can then be used as though it's on your spice rack, sprinkling on any savory dish you wish to.

Dried shitakes that have soaked in warm water to rehydrate become soft enough to puree and **use as a stuffing.** (Save the water you've soaked them in. There's lots of flavor there, too.) To make **meat pinwheels,** spread your pureed shitake mushrooms along with fresh green herbs and a little garlic onto pieces of veal, chicken or turkey breast that you've pounded thin. Roll up the meat and place seam side down on a baking sheet. This creates a meaty shitake roll-up you'll bake whole, like a roast. After it's baked, slice crosswise into 1 inch pinwheels. The more colorful the ingredients you use for stuffing (basil, piquillo peppers, etc.) the more colorful each individual meat pinwheel will be.

11. Zucchini and other summer squash

Zucchini, yellow crookneck squash, pattypan squash and Mexican *calabcitas* are all similar in taste and texture and are all considered "summer squash." Other varieties of summer squash you may see are golden zucchini, romanesco zucchini, eight ball zucchini, yellow straight neck squash, cousa squash and zephyr squash.

What all summer squash have in common that's relevant to HCG is high water content; this means you can eat a *ton* of it on P2. You'll recall that these veggies are so low in carbohydrate, they appear on Tier 1 of our suggested vegetable choices. All summer squash have relatively bland flesh, which will work to our advantage, if we're clever.

Zucchini and summer squash are not everyone's favorite veggie, but they offer a tremendous advantage for P2 cooking: they **become creamy when baked a long time.** If you puree that baked squash, you have the beginnings of a batter.

This **squash batter** is super low in calories and carbs. It doesn't taste like much; you will use it to bulk-up other HCG dishes.

Baked summer squash puree for cake and waffle batter

Yields 1.5 cups batter

— Preheat oven to 375° F degrees.

— Peel and trim the ends from 1.5 pounds fresh summer squash of any kind.
   Yellow crookneck squash works especially well.

— Roughly chop the peeled squash into one-inch chunks.

— Place squash chunks in a heavy pot with a lid (or an oven-safe pan covered with foil).

— Bake covered at 375 degrees for 45 minutes.

— When done, a fork inserted should go through the squash with no resistance.

— Drain off any liquid.

— Puree the baked squash with a food processor or hand mixer, until smooth.

— Optional: Add 2 tsp of a granular alternative natural sweetener

— Optional: Add 1/4 tsp kosher salt.

If you plan to use your batter only in desserts, add 2 tsp of any granular alternative natural sweetener while it's still warm. The sweetener masks any remaining squash flavor and brings out the slight natural sweetness of the squash.

If you keep the summer squash batter naked, you'd add it to savory dishes like a waffle omelet or a cabbage roll. If you add sweetener and cinnamon or cocoa powder, your batter can bulk-up desserts like the **chocolate soufflé mini-cake.** This recipe appears later, under "Searching Precise Recipes Online."

Zucchini and other summer squash may be cut lengthwise and scooped out of their seeds. Once filled and baked you've got a **squash boat with spiced ground meat.** Cinnamon is a spice that works well for both sweet and savory dishes; it pairs especially well with both the squash and the ground meat in a squash boat.

12. Spinach

Throughout this book, one of the ingredients most often mentioned is spinach. When it's raw, spinach makes a beautiful pesto or gourmet salad. When cooked, it's a colorful addition to a meat pinwheel and takes on flavor like curry beautifully. Spinach freezes well, is inexpensive and is fabulous for weight loss.

If you're eating with someone not doing HCG, try preparing the same spinach dish two ways: one intended for Phase 2, one not. For example, **spinach-basil sauté** is a side dish served in some restaurants, with a gorgeous lemon butter in the dish. Few people would be able to refuse it. Without the butter, the dish is perfectly fine for P2.

Begin by cooking down fresh spinach leaves and fresh basil leaves with just enough water or broth to make the greens tender. Use a 5:1 spinach-to-basil ratio. Add several generous squeezes of Meyer lemon juice. Season with smoked maldon salt if you have it, regular sea salt if you don't. Grate fresh nutmeg over the pan, taste and adjust to your liking. Remove your HCG portion from the pan. To make a non-HCG version, add a generous amount of unsalted butter to the pan and incorporate into the hot greens. Serve to non-HCG dining companions.

Spinach has other merits, one of which requires finesse to describe: many of our patients report that spinach whips right through them... so effectively that they notice good weight loss the morning after they've had spinach for dinner. Leafy greens have that effect on a lot of people, especially those who don't eat them often. If your motivation for the diet is waning and you need a good morning result, consider a spinach dish for dinner the night before.

Stir-Fry Featuring Veggies

Let's begin with a sobering reality: it's tough to stir-fry when you cannot fry. Without oil in your pan, you've got to improvise with other cooking liquids. **Consider using as your stir fry liquid:**

1. Fat free chicken broth or stock
2. Unsweetened vinegars like apple cider, raw coconut or rice vinegar
3. Liquid aminos, coconut aminos or tamari, to mimic the flavor of soy sauce
4. A squeeze of fresh lemon, lime or grapefruit juice
5. Fish stock from crab and shrimp shells, fish bones

All of these are clever ways to sauté without oil, and the results can be reasonably good, but liquid in general has a tendency to make things steam rather than get crispy. Here are a couple of tips for stir-frying while on HCG Phase 2.

To minimize steaming, use as little liquid as possible. Use *just enough* liquid to keep things from sticking to the pan. A dryer stir fry will be more crisp.

Second, use a higher heat than you might otherwise. This will encourage browning and minimize steaming.

If you go looking online for HCG recipes, you may see some that some people use a little coconut oil for stir frying on P2. It may be that they have confused MCT oil, which is *derived* from coconut oil, with regular coconut oil. We don't recommend using coconut oil on P2, since the point is to pull the fat from your own body. However, our usual caveat applies: if being able to use a little spray of coconut oil on your pan is the difference between your being able to stick with the diet and giving up, do it.

Rainbow chard with garlic and orange zest

To make Swiss chard with garlic and orange zest, put a few tablespoons of broth or stock in a pan, add a touch of garlic paste until it has incorporated with the broth. Increase heat and sauté chard or any other tender green, like spinach or beet greens, in this garlic broth. Season with smoked sea salt, orange zest and a few red pepper flakes. This dish would be good as a bed of greens for your protein of choice, or as your entire dinner if you don't have many calories left for the day.

Curried spinach with roasted lemon

Curry and lemon both work very well with spinach. To make curried spinach with roasted lemon, thinly slice lemon and roast it in a 425 degree oven until it is soft and golden brown. Squeeze the juice of the roasted lemon into a hot sauté pan, then toss in the roasted lemon pulp. Add your curry powder to bloom in the hot lemon juice. Once you can really smell the curry, add your spinach and sauté until tender, with a lid on pan to create a lemon curry sauce.

Use any curried greens like this one instead of rice as a bed for your proteins. This technique for curry + roasted lemon would bring flavor to a wide variety of seafood, meats and veggies.

Gai-lan and shitake mushrooms with "oyster sauce"

Gai-lan is that platter of broccoli you get at Chinese restaurants that comes drizzled in oyster sauce. It has long stems that are woody and crunchy, with tender leaves at the top. Gai-lan with shitake mushrooms and HCG oyster sauce is a natural for HCG Phase 2.

To emulate oyster sauce, combine coconut aminos as your base, with a little fish sauce in a microwave-safe bowl. Add fresh ginger, a small amount of Swerve or Stevia glycerite and a tiny pinch of xanthan gum or glucomannan to thicken (both optional). Microwave sauce about 30 seconds; as it cools, it should thicken a bit.

Gai-lan takes a while to cook. You may want to microwave it 90 seconds before putting in the skillet. Sauté gai-lan and shitake mushrooms in any broth. Finish the dish with a generous drizzle of your oyster sauce over the sautéed veggies.

Cabbage or konjac noodles with spicy ground meat

Your choices for noodles are shirataki (konjac) noodles and thinly sliced cabbage. Slicing fresh cabbage thinly in your food processor or spiralizer makes longer shreds than buying a bag of cabbage for cole slaw does. Likewise, making shirataki noodles as thin as possible by shaving a yam cake block paper thin in the food processor gives them more the mouth-feel of real noodles. You can use either of both of these things as the "noodles" in your dish.

If you are using shirataki noodles and don't have a full yam cake to work with, the easiest choice is to buy shirataki "angel hair pasta." These thin noodles are more tender than the thicker udon, fettucine or linguine versions they make.

To make **noodles with spicy ground meat**, marinate your shredded cabbage or konjac noodles in coconut aminos, fresh ginger and hot sauce and leave in the fridge at least an hour. Drain most of the marinade, but set aside about 3 tablespoons to serve as your stir-fry liquid.

Heat a few tablespoons of marinade in pan, then add the noodles. Heat noodles until softened. Add ground meat of choice: ground bison, pork tenderloin, chicken breast, etc. (Make sure it's ground, not diced, so you'll distribute the flavor throughout the dish.) Add a little grated onion if you can afford the carbs that day. Stir fry until the meat is cooked through, then remove from heat. Drain any excess liquid and serve.

More Vegetable Dishes

Here are a few more meal ideas that feature vegetables. Any sort of greens will give you a lot of bang for your buck if you're looking for large portion size. Saving leftover soup broth for simmering your greens can be a time-saver.

Baby bok choy simmered in fish broth
Spinach salad with sweet and sour vinaigrette
Kohlrabi cole slaw
Vindaloo curry with eggplant and protein of choice
Blanched Chinese long beans with ginger vinaigrette
Pea vines blanched with fresh mint and ginger

If you've never eaten pea vines or kohlrabi, consider trying them. Both are Tier 2 veggies, so you can have a large portion if you do like them. **Pea vines** are easiest to find in Asian grocery stores, usually in plastic bags. They are the crisp, delicate, curly shoots that grow on pea pods. Pea vines taste very fresh, slightly starchy, slightly sweet. **Kohlrabi** may be found in nearly any market, but often in the section of small baskets with the less popular vegetables.

Kohlrabi is cruciferous; it's the stinky cheese of the vegetable world. It's hard and crunchy, like the thick stem end of broccoli in flavor and texture. If your favorite cheese is Monterey Jack, you probably won't like kohlrabi. If you favor Camembert, you'll probably appreciate kohlrabi's funk. Because it's got dense crunch, eating it raw (as in cole slaw, above) is the way to go.

Pickling veggies for sides and condiments

Cucumbers make good pickles (especially small "pickling cucumbers," which are very firm) but don't stop there. You can pickle **radishes, green tomatoes, bell peppers, celery, cabbage, green beans, kohlrabi, cauliflower, fennel, daikon, ginger, asparagus, mustard greens** and anything else you get your mitts on that's safe for Phase 2. Use the recipe for Refrigerator Pickles later in the book.

Crisp, pickled vegetables make a nice snack, but they're especially valuable as a condiment or a side for your P2 cooking. A piece of plain baked fish can be a bit dismal, but with some **pickled mustard greens** on the side, you've got more variation in taste and texture.

With the refrigerator pickle method, vegetables are not fermented; they have been chilled in a flavorful brine and taken on the flavors in that brine. The good news is that refrigerator pickles are crisp, delicious and ready to eat in as little as three hours. The bad news is that they last only a couple of weeks in the fridge.

The boilerplate recipe for refrigerator pickles in the "Quick Bites" chapter is for **half sour pickles.** These are crisp, refreshing, slightly briny pickles that are less sour than Kosher dills are. You can monkey with the recipe to create more sour, sweet, briny or spicy pickles; monkeying with it is the point.

Our recipe for refrigerator pickles includes a long list of aromatics: the herbs, spices, fruits and other elements that you will combine to give your pickles the flavor profile you're shooting for. Below are a few examples of how you can play with aromatics to personalize your refrigerator pickles.

Flavor ideas for pickling veggies

...Cloves, sweetener and one Thai chile = **sweet and sour pickle with a little heat**

...Dill, allspice, celery seed, mustard seed and peppercorns = **traditional deli pickle**

...Fresh ginger, lemon, lime or grapefruit slices + fresh mint = **clean, refreshing pickle**

...Fresh garlic and jalapeños = **savory and spicy pickle**

...Fresh turmeric and orange slices = **earthy pickle, bright orange color**

...Lime, kaffir lime leaves, lemongrass = **subtle, Thai herb pickle**

...Curry powder, sweetener, allspice, fennel = **curried sweet pickle**

The ginger/citrus/mint pickles above are real MVPs. Even people who say they don't like pickles usually love these. They're not sour or acidic, just fresh and crisp with a refined flavor profile.

Also really delicious are the curried bread and butter (sweet and sour) pickles. They're a gourmet version of the pickle chips of your childhood. As you can imagine, they are fabulous chopped into a relish for tuna salad.

You might also make **homemade pickled ginger** to go with your sashimi. The pink, store-bought pickled ginger contains sugar, but yours would not. Use a vegetable peeler to shave very thin pieces from a finger of fresh ginger. Sweeten some plain rice vinegar with stevia glycerite or other alternative natural sweetener that dissolves well. Add a big pinch of salt. (Be certain your rice vinegar is not "seasoned rice vinegar" or "sushi vinegar," because both have sugar.) Marinate the ginger in the vinegar mixture at least one hour. Save that marinade for some other dish; it will be a sweet and sour ginger vinaigrette that tastes fabulous.

Japanese cucumber salad (*sunomono*) is one thing you could do with that leftover ginger marinade. Combine rice vinegar + sweetener + a little salt (or use your pickled ginger marinade). You'll probably need to taste your brine multiple times to achieve the sweet/sour balance you most enjoy.

Thinly slice tender cucumbers like Persian or English hothouse cucumbers and submerge them in the marinade. Chopped, fresh mint is a delicious addition, though it's not the traditional Japanese rendition. Leave your thinly sliced cucumbers in the pickling brine for at least 30 minutes, though about two hours is best. This is all the time it takes for the flavor to transfer to the cucumbers if they've been thinly sliced. Drain well and save the liquid.

How to Make Egg Whites Palatable

Egg whites make a very useful breakfast on P2. They are filling, use very few of your day's calories, have a terrific protein density score (12) and they're a snap to make in the microwave. Two egg whites microwaved for about 1 minute, 10 seconds turn out fluffy. If you use a disposable bowl, you've got no cleanup.

That said, plain egg whites are not scrumptious. They beat a growling belly, though, and there are some ways to work creatively with them. Try **leftovers chopped up in your egg whites**, like a mashed chicken meatball or a couple of mushrooms or garlic spinach. You can't use butter, but you can use smoked salt and pepper and you can use hot sauce. Sambal olek [Indonesian chili paste] is good on egg whites, as is yuzu hot sauce. Your homemade HCG ketchup will make egg whites taste amazing.*

* Amazing is relative.

An egg white meal is also a good time to use an ingredient you really like but can only eat a tiny bit of while on HCG. For example, **half an artichoke heart** is a delicious addition to baked egg whites. You can't eat much artichoke heart (Tier 3 — only as a treat) but this addition could make your egg whites palatable. The same goes for ingredients you might ordinarily put in an omelette, but can't have much of on HCG, like a few **caramelized onions** or a bit of **smoked salmon.**

Another example of using a special, tasty ingredient for your egg whites is making **wood-fired piquillo pepper sauce.** Buy a jar or tin of wood-fired piquillo peppers, which usually come packed in water, not oil. Puree with a little salt, lemon zest, 1/2 clove garlic and fresh herbs. The resulting sauce will be very thick and flavorful. Thin it with a little water if you want to stretch the sauce, then cook it down by simmering for about 10 minutes. Just a couple teaspoons of piquillo pepper sauce will pep up your egg whites in a major way. The sauce would also be great on bland fish, on asparagus, broccoli, Brussels sprouts, cauliflower and such.

If you are willing to use more of your calories at breakfast in exchange for a yummy meal, you could make an **inside-out breakfast sandwich.** Microwave one egg white in a ramekin, then repeat. You will now have two cooked egg whites that are flat and round. Remove from ramekins and pat dry; these will be your "bread." Your filling might be leftover rotisserie chicken or pork tenderloin with "honey mustard." To make **sausage patties** for your inside-out breakfast sandwich, grind raw meat with fresh herbs like sage and dried spices like fennel then form into rounds and cook on a cast iron pan.

Using egg whites as the *outside* of a sandwich is messy, but it's an example of a mental hack for HCG. Do things you wouldn't ordinarily do!

A Course in Miracle Noodles

Shirataki Noodles are Japanese noodles made from the konjac root. They are sometimes referred to generically as "miracle noodles" in discussions of HCG cooking, but Miracle Noodle is actually a brand name of shirataki noodle.

Because the konjac root is a resistant starch, our body does not digest it fully, thus these noodles are extremely low in carbs and calories. They don't taste like much, and they are not as tender as ordinary noodles are, but you can use shirataki noodles to make your dishes more filling, which is a huge help during Phase 2. We have a few tricks to offer.

Your shirataki noodles come in a brine, so you'll need to rinse them well. If you're using them in hot soup, they're ready to go after rinsing. If you want to use them for a stir fry, you can boil or microwave them to soften a bit, or can cook them alone in a dry sauce pan to make them less slimy. This trick works! Frankly, shirataki noodles never get super tender, the way an egg pasta noodle would, but they multi-task really well for P2.

One clever strategy for making these noodles tender is to buy your shirataki in block form rather than noodle form, if you have access to an Asian market. The product is usually Japanese and will typically be labeled "yam cake." You can then use your food processor to slice this brick into very thin ribbons. You'll produce wide noodles that are more tender than the packaged shirataki noodles are.

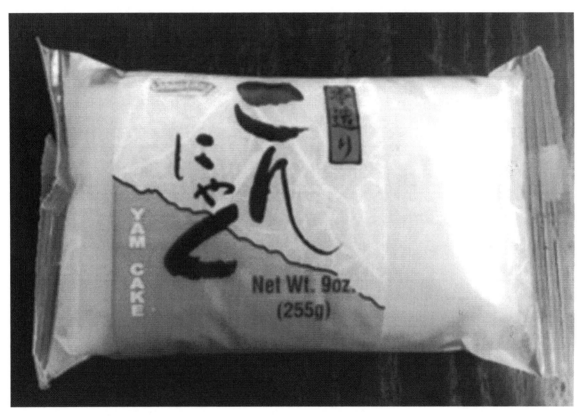

Shirataki as a block or "yam cake" looks like this. You can slice this extra thin in your food processor to make your noodles more tender to bite.. You might also puree yam cake to create a porridge. Add a flavor extract, like coconut.

You can marinate shirataki noodles in **coconut aminos,** which tastes like a sweet soy sauce. The noodles don't *entirely* absorb flavors, but marinating does help.

Another idea: you may transform *any* shirataki product, block or noodles, into the **texture of rice** by blitzing it in your food processor. Make it the texture of porridge by pureeing and adding a little water.

Use shirataki rice to **make dishes more filling,** the way you would use Hamburger Helper: add it to your stew, meatballs, soup, chili, stuffed peppers, cabbage rolls and such to increase portion size without adding calories.

You can even add pureed shirataki noodles to a dessert like a mug cake, protein shake or gelatin squares. It may seem odd to add texture but no flavor to a dish, but we think it's kind of clever — feeling full on just 500-800 calories requires strategy.

If you don't mind the chew of shirataki rice, here's a funky breakfast or dessert idea for P2. Let's call it **cinnamon rice jumble.**

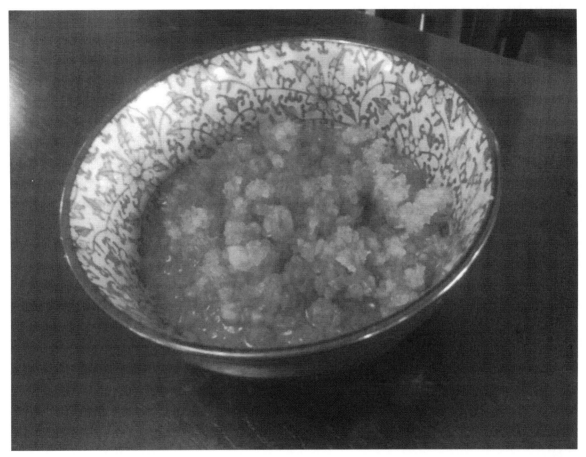

Photo: Dana Falk

Will cinnamon rice jumble rock your world? Not unless you are quite hungry, but it's extremely filling and that's a virtue. It tastes like a sweet, lumpy porridge. This recipe for a big bowl o' jumble is only 21 calories.

245

Cinnamon Rice Jumble

Two packages (7-8 oz apiece) shirataki noodles, any kind
2 tbs brewed spice tea (chai tea, orange spice, cinnamon tea, etc.)
10 drops flavored stevia glycerite
Good quality cinnamon
Pinch salt

— Drain and rinse the shirataki noodles.

— Place drained shirataki in a blender or food processor. Puree.

— Add 2 tbs strongly brewed spice tea.
  It will not look as though you're adding enough liquid, but the shirataki itself gives off liquid when heated.

— Add a large pinch of salt and up to 10 drops of flavored stevia glycerite: French vanilla, cinnamon-vanilla, maple and chai spice flavors all work well.

— Add a rounded 1/4 tsp of the best quality cinnamon you've got.

— Puree again. Mixture will never become entirely smooth.

— Heat 1 minute 15 seconds in microwave.

— Sprinkle additional cinnamon on top and serve.

Is this recipe for *one* serving of cinnamon rice jumble or two? The whole damn thing is only 21 calories so it's totally up to you. Will cinnamon rice jumble remind you of the creamy, aromatic basmati rice pudding you've had at your favorite Indian restaurant? No, but it sure feels nice to have a dessert or breakfast porridge that's sweet and filling when you're on Phase 2.

Unlike some of the ingredients we've described in *HCG for Foodies*, shirataki noodle products are inexpensive. The shelf stable versions cost a bit more than the refrigerated versions do, but they come in a wider variety of options.

There are many brands of shirataki to consider. One is called **Shirakiku**; it's in the refrigerated section of stores that carry Asian foods. Shirakiku brand has noodles that resemble angel hair pasta, yakisoba, and udon in thickness, as well as the block or "yam cake" form. Look also for **Pasta Zero** in the refrigerated section of mainstream markets.

The shelf stable versions often come in more shapes than the refrigerated versions do. **Miracle Noodle** for example offers angel hair pasta, spaghetti, fettucine, ziti and rice shapes, at the time of this writing. The thicker cuts, like their ziti, are very dense; not as pleasing a mouth feel as the thinner cuts, like the fettucine, in our opinion.

Vitacost's house brand, ***Shirataki Pasta*** and Thrive Market's house brand, ***Wonder Noodles*** (both online) are excellent. Both of these are tender enough to do good things with. Attention foodie nerds: the Vitacost "fettucine" noodles are actually the width of linguine; just right for preparing with some seafood.

Don't accidentally buy "Tofu Shirataki Noodles." These are soy, so they're more carby and caloric. Also, soy contains strong phytoestrogens. These are plant molecules that look a lot like estrogen and have an estrogen-like effect on the body, such as fluid retention and weight gain. Phytoestrogens may be helpful if your estrogen is low — talk to your doctor if that's the case — but while on HCG, soy products are not recommended. This includes plain or flavored tofu, soy sauce, edamame, tempeh, veggie burgers or sausage patties made with "textured soy protein" as well as all tofu-based shirataki noodles.

Fish and Shellfish Dishes

Many of the foods that are best-suited to HCG are fish and shellfish. Shellfish come in several forms: *crustaceans* like crab, lobster, shrimp and crawfish and *mollusks* like clams, oysters, scallops and mussels. Though these foods are not equally high in protein density, you'll find that many of the foods you can have a large serving of while on HCG are fish and shellfish.

Definitely take a look at the seafood section of a good market to see if there's anything not in your usual rotation that would be worth a try while on HCG. **Halibut cheeks** are a good example of a seafood that's delicious but often forgotten. Halibut cheeks look and taste like huge scallops — slightly sweet, tender and a little stringy — but they have much better numbers for P2 than scallops do. When they're in season, man they're good.

Research protein scores to inform your choices. Let's say you like both shrimp and salmon quite a bit. Shrimp's protein density score is about 8. That's over 4, so it's great. Salmon's score is 3.65, which is passable, not ideal. (Makes logical sense, because salmon is oily.) You can eat both shrimp and salmon on P2, but your choice would be between a large serving of shrimp and a small serving of salmon.

Here are some ideas for P2 cooking that feature fish and shellfish:

Sashimi grade ahi tuna

Ahi tuna (or any other lean fish that is sold extremely fresh) would work for sashimi. **Halibut** is good. **Octopus** is good. **Yellowtail** works but is higher fat, so you can eat less of it. Don't choose fatty tuna, eel, herring, sardines, anchovies, sea bass and mackerel, which are all oily. Avoid them on Phase 2 but look forward to eating them again on Phase 3.

For a dipping sauce that mimics the **ponzu sauce** you'd have with sashimi, start with coconut aminos as your soy sauce, add a little lime juice, a little rice vinegar, a little water and a few drops of your alternative sweetener, like Sweet Leaf stevia drops or Now Foods Better Stevia glycerite.

It's tough to make **tuna poke** without the use of sesame oil, but it's worth a try: chopped green onions, coconut aminos, a little hot sauce and a little alternative natural sweetener like All-u-lose honey syrup will emulate poke fairly well. A little shake of sesame seeds for garnish won't kill you, but do avoid sesame oil.

TIP: Coconut aminos, tamari and Bragg's liquid aminos are all P2 substitutes for soy sauce. Liquid aminos are the saltiest of the three and **coconut aminos** are the sweetest. For making poke or teriyaki, coconut aminos would be your best bet.

Grilled swordfish

Putting swordfish or another sturdy fish like marlin or tuna on a panini grill gives you some flavor to work with. To make **charred herbed swordfish with vinaigrette**, salt and pepper the fish on both sides (use hot pepper flakes rather than black pepper, if you like). Finely chop your fresh green herbs of choice, perhaps cilantro, and use the natural moisture of the filet to dredge it on both sides in the herbs. The herbs will turn brown when you grill them, but they provide flavor.

You will not marinate the fish in a dressing with MCT oil, because the high heat of the panini grill would make it smoke. Instead, make a simple **MCT cilantro-lime vinaigrette** to drizzle on the finished, grilled fish. Use chopped, fresh cilantro (or other green herb) + rice vinegar + lime juice + MCT oil + sweetener such as stevia glycerite. Shake well. Place charred herb fish on a bed of greens and dress with your herb vinaigrette.

Vietnamese prawn noodle bowl

Shirataki noodles + shredded romaine lettuce + chopped fresh mint or Thai basil (optional) + grilled prawns with grated garlic + lime vinaigrette = **Vietnamese prawn noodle bowl.** Your **lime vinaigrette** = fresh lime juice + lime zest + rice vinegar + MCT oil + stevia glycerite.

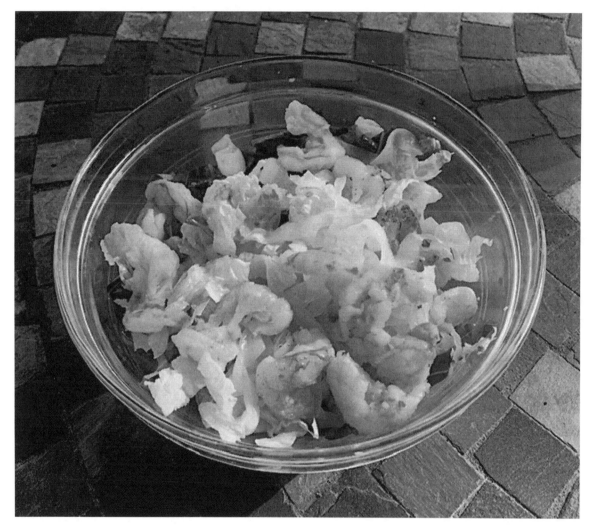

Photo: Dana Falk

Vietnamese prawn noodle bowl = shredded romaine and shirataki noodles dressed in zesty lime vinaigrette, then topped with garlic prawns. Would be even better with chopped mint or basil, but already tastes great.

Rinse noodles well, then place in a medium hot pan until they are dry. Shred lettuce. Chop herbs, if using. Slice prawns in half lengthwise and place in a non-stick skillet. Use a microplane to grate one clove garlic on the prawns. Add a teaspoon of water or broth if they are sticking and cook until lightly browned.

Make dressing: shake some fresh-squeezed lime juice and lots of zest, rice vinegar and MCT oil in an airtight container. Add a few drops stevia glycerite to taste and shake again.

Toss noodles, shredded lettuce and herbs (if using). Dress the noodles and greens lightly with lime vinaigrette. Top with cooked garlic prawns. Drizzle a little additional dressing on prawns and enjoy.

Baked filet of sole (and other flat fish)

Dover sole, petrale sole, rex sole, sand dabs and flounder are all types of flat fish. These all have a delicate taste and texture; they're good for people who don't love the taste of fish but want a protein they can eat a lot of.
Sole and other flat fish usually come in thin, delicate fillets in the fresh seafood case. These are not generally expensive fish. The fact that they are thin filets is helpful if you don't love fish, because you can purposely overcook them if you want, to assure they won't be mushy.

Rex sole is sometimes sold as a whole fish and is considered one of the tastiest of the flat fish. By contrast, Trader Joe's sells packages of frozen Dover sole filets that would be easy to have on hand.

For **baking filet of sole,** which is delicate in flavor and texture, a marinade is not really necessary, nor is an assertive spice mix, though some people like to use blackened spice mix to create a Cajun favor. A little good quality salt, some grated fresh ginger and some citrus zest should do it for prep. Allowing it to remain in the fridge for at least an hour after you've rubbed it with the salt, ginger and citrus will result in a more flavorful dish. (If you want to go uptown, make it a crust of lavender salt and orange zest.)

Preheat the oven to 375° F degrees for a relatively moist fish or 400 degrees if you're purposely trying to dry it out. Line a cookie sheet with parchment paper, place the fish filets in the oven and cook to your preferred doneness. The internal temperature should be 145° F if you want the filet of sole to be moist.

Crab cakes or shrimp cakes

Pre-packaged crab meat is pretty darn good if you drain it well. Sometimes you'll see it in cans, other times in plastic tubs in the refrigerated section. Be careful not to buy the hunks of *imitation* crab meat used in some sushi; these contain starches. Shrimp may be less luxurious than crab is, but it purees so perfectly for shrimp cakes and they hold together better than crab cakes do.

Making **crab or shrimp cakes** without mayonnaise, bread crumbs or oil for frying is a challenge, but it can be done. The recipe that follows is imprecise; you will need to tinker with the flavors and texture to your satisfaction. Since crab and shrimp are both ingredients you can eat a lot of, make a large batch once your version tastes good.

Crab or Shrimp Cakes

In general, shrimp cakes hold together better than crab cakes do. Remember, these have no mayo in them and no bread crumbs on them, so they will not be as tender or crisp as regular crab cakes are. These function more like a flavorful bite for a nori wrap or lettuce wrap.

1 pound fresh crab or shrimp

Rounded 1/3 cup diced celery

1/4 cup diced red, yellow or orange bell pepper

1/4 cup finely chopped onion

2 tbs fat-free chicken broth

1/4 tsp salt

1 clove garlic

Up to 1 tsp lemon zest

2 tbs chopped fresh parsley or basil

1/8 tsp Old Bay Seasoning - OR - 3/4 tsp minced lemongrass

Optional:

2 tbs cooked, mashed radish or cauliflower

Red chili flakes or diced hot peppers to taste

If using crab: pat meat dry and set aside.

If using raw shrimp: Separate 1/3 pound of the shrimp meat and chop roughly. Puree the remaining 2/3 pound of raw shrimp in food processor.

— Roughly chop the celery, onion and bell pepper. Add the garlic clove and pulse in a food processor.

— Heat broth in a skillet, then add chopped veggies and garlic. Add salt and lemongrass or Old Bay and cook until soft.

— Remove from heat and place in mixing bowl. If using mashed radish or cauliflower, add now.

— Add lemon zest and fresh chopped herbs. If using hot pepper flakes or peppers, add now. Mix to combine.

— Add the crab or shrimp meat and incorporate well. (If using shrimp, add both the pureed and the chopped shrimp meat.)

— Refrigerate the mixture at least 30 mins, so it will be more sturdy.

— Preheat oven to 425° F degrees.

— After 30 min, form mixture into patties about 1/2 inch thick and 2 1/2 inches wide.

— Arrange on aluminum foil or parchment-lined cookie sheet, with plenty of space between them, as flipping can be tricky. (Depending upon how many patties you've formed, you may need to bake in two batches.)

— Bake crab or shrimp cakes at 425° F degrees for 10-12 mins, then flip. Continue baking until lightly browned on second side, another 2-3 mins.

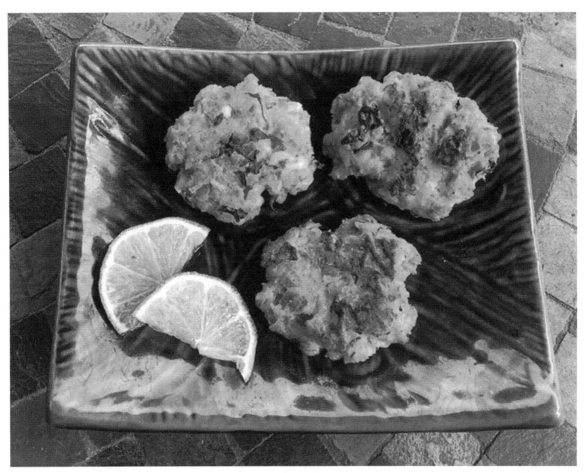

Photo: Dana Falk

Shrimp cakes made with basil, red bell pepper and Old Bay seasoning, which gives them an orange cast. These are good hot, as an entree, or room temperature, in a lettuce wrap or nori wrap.

Crab and shrimp cakes may be frozen individually after they have cooled. You then bake to reheat them as you would any frozen food. You'll have a go-to dish that's perfect with a side salad. If you make your crab cakes all the same weight, you'll know what to enter in your tracking app each time.

Calamari

You may see calamari (squid) sold as ringlets, as the whole cleaned squid (which is a long tube) or pounded flat, into steaks. Calamari is mild in flavor, it's sturdy for travel and is really healthy — it has terrific protein density score for Phase 2. People love or hate calamari. If you love it, or can learn to like it, that's an advantage on HCG. In Asian markets you can sometimes find **dried cuttlefish or squid** in the snack section, too, but read the label; some contain sugar or MSG.

In the US, calamari is often prepared breaded and pan fried, served with lemon wedges, but in the Mediterranean you'll find **calamari marinated in citrus, herbs and capers and char-grilled at high heat.** In Italian cuisine, calamari may be **braised in a spicy, tomato-based broth.** Both the Italian and Mediterranean preparations would work well for HCG Phase 2. If you can avoid breading the calamari with ground Melba toast or other crackers, you'll have more calories and carbs left for other things.

If you decide to give **sautéed calamari** a whirl, cooking it in a covered saucepan will give you tender results. Your liquid could be the juice of 1/2 lemon and several tablespoons liquid from a can of diced tomatoes. Add fresh thyme, a little garlic, a good amount of salt, and you've got an interesting and filling dish that you could eat a lot of.

Some people prefer to eat sautéed calamari chilled, on a **seafood salad.** Try slicing Belgian endive thinly instead of using lettuce greens. Dress the endive lightly in an MCT lemon vinaigrette, then top with chilled shrimp, crab, calamari, scallops — whatever you have on hand. Another drizzle of the lemon vinaigrette on the seafood to finish.

Crawfish tails

Crawfish (also called crayfish or crawdads) are more flavorful than shrimp; they seem to have a natural balance of sweetness and saltiness all their own. They look like mini lobsters and usually come in their shells, but occasionally you can find bags of just crawfish meat in the frozen section. If you can find this, grab it! Crawfish has a terrific protein density score of 15. Occasionally, frozen crawfish come packaged in a butter sauce, so look closely before stocking up.

Try preparing **crawfish gumbo** in a dutch oven with a lid. Begin by toasting blackened spice mix, gumbo file spice or a Cajun spice mix at the bottom of the pan at low heat. Add diced green bell pepper, diced celery and canned, fire roasted tomato, including the liquid. Then add the crawfish and any other protein or veggies you'd like to use up. A small amount of chopped onion will help, if you have the carbs to spare. Chicken or turkey breast works as an add-in, as does pork tenderloin, but the briny flavor of the crawfish should be the star of this dish.

Increase the heat to medium-low, replace the lid and simmer at least 30 minutes. Using the lid will help the dish create its own sauce. If you want this to be thick like a gumbo, leave as is. If you want it to be a thinner soup, add some fat-free broth.

Serve with collard greens or mustard greens if you've got them. If you want a crawfish dish that would be eaten in a radicchio cup or lettuce wrap, drain the liquid from your gumbo and save in the freezer for some future dish.

Crawfish meat is very tasty. You may find that plain crawfish meat that's been cooked in salty water is all you need. Chill it, throw in a zipper bag and be on your way.

Ceviche

Ceviche is a raw seafood cocktail that's been cooked by the acid of the citrus juice it marinates in. Cut your seafood into bite size pieces. **Scallops, tuna, firm white fish like halibut, prawns, squid and octopus** are all good for making ceviche. Add chopped cucumber and/or radish. Add finely chopped jalapeño if you'd like and a pinch of good salt. Thinly sliced onion is traditional, but try to either (a) use just a tiny bit of onion or (b) keep the onion in big pieces while the ceviche marinates, then remove the pieces before serving.

Your marinade may be lemon or lime juice. Classic ceviche has a little sugar, but a squeeze of orange or a pinch of alternative natural sweetener will substitute for sugar in yours. Remove from the marinade when the fish is no longer raw. Drain well.

Traditionally, ceviche is served in a footed glass and garnished with avocado, chopped tomato and fresh cilantro or parsley. Avocado doesn't work for HCG Phase 2, but it's back in your life once you're on Phase 3. For now, garnish with fresh herbs and a little fresh tomato.

Fresh oysters

Fresh oysters are reasonably good for P2; they have a protein density of 4. They're mentioned here mostly because they make a good appetizer choice if you have to eat at a fancy restaurant while on P2. Use a squeeze of lemon instead of the vinaigrette that comes with oysters, because it usually has sugar.

At home, you may cook oysters on the grill, still on the half shell. If you have a smoker, these are a natural. If you buy them smoked, check the ingredient list for sugar and soybean oil. Smoked oysters have a lot of flavor, so just a little bit used as an ingredient in a gumbo, for example, would be valuable.

Cioppino and Bouillabaisse

Cioppino and bouillabaisse are both soups that contain big pieces of fish or shellfish, cooked gently in a savory broth. Some regard them stews, actually, because they're more about the seafood than the soup base. Cioppino and bouillabaisse call for the same cooking process, so we'll consider them together.

Cioppino is made with a spicy, tomato-infused broth. It usually has clams, mussels, crab and a few pieces of fish such as salmon. Bouillabaisse is made with a fish stock (think broth made with leftover crab shells, prawn shells and lobster shells) and it usually has chunks of firm white fish, like cod, orange roughy, red snapper, rockfish or halibut. Both are delicious, stretch your calories for the day, and could be served to other people without tipping them off that you're eating carefully.

Begin **cioppino** with a quart of fat-free chicken broth. Add about 1/4 cup of strained tomatoes or diced, canned tomatoes and about 1/2 tsp kosher salt. (Be certain it's kosher salt, not table salt, or it will be too salty.) Add about 1 tsp of diced hot peppers or some hot sauce. Grate in some garlic, throw in a little diced onion, some diced celery and you've got a basic cioppino broth. If you have some **fresh fennel** to add, big bonus. Heat broth, then turn down to a simmer for about 20 minutes. Add whatever fish and shellfish you'd like and simmer on low until the seafood is cooked through. Turn off the heat and let the soup sit off heat before eating; the flavors will deepen.

Bouillabaisse begins with a quart of fat-free chicken broth. Add leftover crustacean shells if you have them. Add about 1 - 1.5 tsp saffron, a little diced onion, a little grated garlic and 1/2 tsp kosher salt. Heat broth, then turn down to a simmer for about 20 minutes. Add chunks of raw fish, 1-2 inches in size. Simmer on low until the seafood is cooked through, then remove from heat. As with cioppino, allowing the bouillabaisse to sit after it has simmered only makes it taste better.

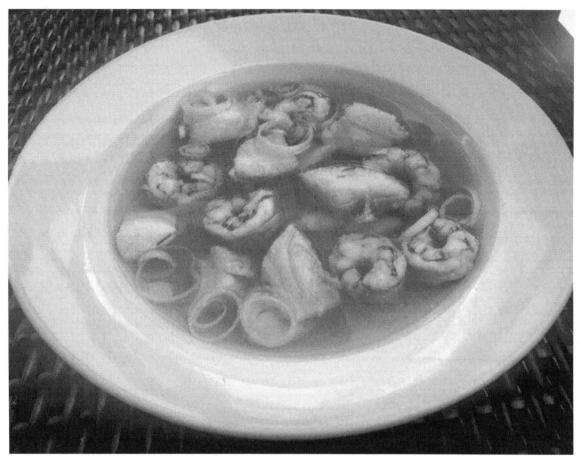

Photo: Dana Falk

A simple bouillabaisse of fresh codfish and prawns is simmered with thinly sliced leek rings, for flavor. Saffron makes fat free chicken broth taste much more complex and makes it look beautiful.

Cioppino and bouillabaisse are both good ways to use up little bits of ingredients you have around: a little celery that needs to be used up, a little chunk of halibut, a few leftover shrimp and some kale? Toss it all in.

Though both these soups are about simmering raw seafood in a flavorful broth so that the fish and the broth will bring out the best in each other, it's fine to just use what you have, even if it's already cooked. Cioppino and bouillabaisse both freeze well.

Orange roughy baked with orange zest

There's no reason you can't be playful with your menu even when suffering. Orange roughy baked with orange zest is a natural. Orange roughy is a firm fish that you can find in the market already filleted. Take your filets and rub them with the zest of an orange, flaky sea salt and some fresh tarragon or other fresh herb. Place in a ziploc bag and refrigerate for at least an hour.

When ready to cook, bake at 350 degrees in a parchment or foil packet with a little squeeze of the orange you zested and more fresh tarragon. The result will be tender, steamed fish infused with orange flavor. If you'd prefer it to brown and be less tender, bake on a cookie sheet instead of in a packet. Orange roughy is also firm enough to be cooked on a grill.

Fresh prawns

Prawns are the Hall of Fame shortstop in your HCG diet — they can field anything that comes their way. Bake or sauté them. Keep them whole, dice or puree them.

Here are a few prawn dishes to try:

— Curried prawns garnished with starfruit

— Lemon garlic prawns over cauliflower rice or zucchini noodles

— Lemongrass-ginger prawns charred on the grill

— Prawns stewed in garam masala with a little tomato

— Raw prawns pureed become a "dumpling" filling for steamed Napa cabbage

— Toss raw prawns into your hot and sour soup and let them cook in the broth

— Slice an overcooked prawn lengthwise and use it to stabilize a wobbly table

Prawns are so versatile. A tip for making them as flavorful as possible: **roast prawns in their shell.** You can buy them with or without heads, deveined or not, just be certain they still have their shells if you're game for extra work in exchange for extra flavor.

De-vein prawns with the shell still on by running a sharp knife along the back and scraping out the dark matter with the point of your knife. Toss them in simple spices— perhaps a little celery salt, some minced lemongrass or some grated nutmeg, then roast prawns at high heat, about 425° F degrees. Keep an eye on them. When they start to look pinkish-orange, flip them. Just a minute or so more and they're done.

It's not necessary to go to this trouble for roasted prawns if you don't want to. Trader Joe's sells **Argentine Red Shrimp** in the frozen food section that have been shelled and cleaned. Despite being sold frozen, they are sweet, tender and delicious when cooked.

Prawns are nice enough to serve to guests. You can offer prawn cocktail as an appetizer or bring it for a potluck and no one would guess you're on a special diet. You can buy a humongous tray of plain, boiled prawns at a warehouse store. If you've made HCG cocktail sauce [below] that's great. If not, put out cocktail sauce from a jar for others to enjoy and eat your own prawns plain or with a squeeze of lemon.

HCG-friendly ketchup and cocktail sauce

You'll need strained tomatoes or marinara sauce to make ketchup and cocktail sauce, so find the lowest carbohydrate versions you can. **Pomi strained tomatoes** are lower in carbohydrate than most. They come in boxes rather than cans, so you needn't transfer leftovers to a plastic container. **Rao's marinara sauce** is also a high quality product and is lower carb than most.

These are not products that you'll see in many published HCG recipes, because tomato sauce has more carbs than whole tomatoes do, but bear in mind that this ketchup and cocktail sauce are condiments you'll use just a dab of. A little HCG ketchup in your cooked ground turkey gives you the beginnings of a **Sloppy Joe.** Serving a little cocktail sauce with jumbo prawns gives you a **shrimp cocktail** to be proud of. These sauces are not meant to be major ingredients, they are mood enhancers.

HCG Ketchup = Strained tomato or marinara + apple cider vinegar + sweetener + salt + (recommended) nutmeg + (optional) onion powder.

HCG Barbecue Sauce = add a couple drops liquid smoke + dash of paprika + dash cinnamon to ketchup recipe above. Optional: few drops worcestershire sauce.

HCG Cocktail Sauce = Strained tomato + salt + crushed celery seed + a little bottled horseradish + a little tabasco. Optional: few drops worcestershire sauce.

Ordinarily, barbecue sauce and cocktail sauce contain worcestershire sauce, which has molasses, sugar and tamarind as ingredients. Leave worcestershire out unless you're willing to use just a dash; it has a very distinctive flavor and does make a difference.

Cook down your sauce in a pan by starting at medium heat, then reducing to low heat once the sauce begins to bubble. Allow to simmer very gently for 10-15 minutes, stirring and tinkering with the balance of flavors. Your sauce will thicken and the flavors will develop. Cool finished sauce. Refrigerate some and freeze the rest.

Quick Bite Ideas

Biltong or Jerky

If you're in the mood for something chewy, **sugar-free beef jerky and biltong** (dried meat) can be quite satisfying. Beef jerky used to be very difficult to find sugar-free, but the demand for keto products has changed that, baby. Consider these store-bought options:

Brand	Product	Grams of fat per ounce
People's Choice	Carne Seca	2.5 grams
Ayoba	Biltong	2.5 grams
Keto Carne	Beef Jerky	2.5 grams
Stryve	Biltong slices (not sticks)	2 grams
Tillamook	Zero sugar beef jerky slices (not sticks or sausages)	1.5 grams
Jack Links	Zero sugar beef jerky	1.5 grams

HCG purists may disagree with jerky and biltong as snack options on Phase 2, but let's do the math. Try a protein density calculation for Tillamook Zero Sugar Beef Jerky, for example. If you recall, the formula for choosing proteins is this:

Protein grams
————————— = **Protein density = How good for you on P2**
Fat + carb grams

For each one ounce serving, the Tillamook product has 14 grams protein, 1.5 grams fat and 0 grams carbohydrate.

14 divided by (1.5 + 0)
= 14 divided by 1.5
= 9.33 protein density (Better than prawns!)
= Damn good snack choice for HCG

As you compare brands (there are far more than appear above) just be sure it's biltong slices or sugar free jerky you're considering (which are ultra lean) rather than a meat stick or sausage (which is soft and fatty, inside a casing).

Making jerky yourself in a low oven or food dehydrator is one way to assure that it's lean meat and that it's sugar-free. There's a detailed recipe in the section "Homemade Jerky." Top round beef and bison sirloin are extremely lean meats, so they make jerky that's tough as shoe leather, but hey, it's nice to have a chewy snack safe for P2.

Smoked oysters, mussels, clams, scallops, trout

This snack may require legwork on your part, as some smoked fish and mollusks are made with soybean oil and sugar — but some are not, and they're delicious. Smoked mollusks and fish may sometimes be found online, vacuum-packed without oil. Local smokehouses and fish markets often have their own house-made smoked fish. Some classic New York style delis offer smoked whitefish, chubs, sturgeon or trout.

Even a fish that's more oily than what you'd ordinarily eat on HCG Phase 2, like sturgeon, can have flavor potential for P2 cooking. Smoked seafood has so much flavor you can use just a tiny bit of it. For example, putting a little bit of smoked whitefish in your MCT oil salad dressing would make it taste like the anchovies in a Caesar salad dressing.

If you are the kind of person who would find it difficult to use a tiny bit of smoked fish, just for flavor, then skip it. There's a section later in the book that helps people understand how to factor their personality into their food choices. It's called "Personal Insights Useful for Weight Loss."

Dehydrated kale and other veggie chips
Kale is sturdy enough to dry well in a low oven or food dehydrator. This is where your trips to ethnic markets will pay off, as you may have delicious spice mixes like **Ethiopian berbere, Kashmiri masala or Middle Eastern Ras al Hanout** to play with. **Dried lemon zest and dried mint** are also nice for making dried kale. Without oil, your dried kale will not be deliciously crisp and tender like fried kale chips are, but it may still hit the spot. If you're in need of hippie street cred, there's nothing better.

Tuna or turkey salad with MCT vinaigrette
The vinaigrette is key. **"Honey" mustard vinaigrette** = cider vinegar + your MCT oil for the day + a few drops stevia glycerite + about 2 tsp mustard + a little salt. For the most authentic tasting honey mustard, rather than sweetening with stevia glycerite, order **Choc Zero's caramel syrup or All-u-lose honey syrup** online. You may also add fresh herbs like thyme, fennel or dill fronds if you'd like.

Shake up your vinaigrette and use it to moisten 1-2 cans of tuna packed in water or some leftover, cubed turkey or chicken breast. Toss in some chopped bell pepper and celery for crunch. It's a blazing fast meal that's quite filling because it's so high in protein.

Some people experience gastrointestinal upset if they take all of their MCT oil for the day in one dose. If that's true for you, use enough tuna or turkey with your dressing that you can make two separate meals of it. Remember: if you share your vinaigrette made with someone who is not accustomed to MCT oil, it could blow right through them. Thus, your HCG tuna or turkey salad has potential as a practical joke and as a high protein meal.

Obviously, this meal is stone cold simple, but a lot of patients tell us that it's important to their round of HCG. Tuna and turkey salad really give you a full belly. When made flavorful with a vinaigrette, it's awfully useful to have on hand.

Canned, roasted chicken breast

The key is *roasted* canned chicken; it has a much nicer flavor than ordinary canned chicken breast does (although plain old canned chicken, as long as it is entirely breast meat packed in water, is excellent for HCG Phase 2 in the nutritional sense). **Wild Planet organic, roasted chicken breast** in a can is doggone good and it comes in a pull-top can so it travels well.

Some people say that eating a can of chicken makes them feel less deprived than eating a can of plain tuna does. If you didn't have any vinaigrette and had to eat one of these right out of the can, you'd likely prefer the roasted chicken; it's more moist.

Cold seared tuna dipped in MCT vinaigrette

Snacks on HCG are often leftovers: a couple of **curried prawns wrapped in a sheet of nori,** a couple of **lamb kofta you wrap in butter lettuce,** or in this case, some **ahi tuna you seared the day before, dipped in your homemade lemon vinaigrette.** Using leftovers as snacks is an efficient approach, since you have already assured that each of these nibbles is safe for P2.

Turkey breast with cranberry sauce

The deli case of some grocery stores has cooked, fresh turkey breast. We're not referring to the thinly sliced turkey *sandwich meat*, but a whole cooked turkey breast. Some grocery stores even sell **whole, roasted turkey breasts** in the same heated display case as the meatloaf and the roasted chickens.

A thick slice of roasted turkey breast, skin removed, tastes quite good; even better with a quick cranberry sauce. **Quick HCG Cranberry sauce** = 3/4 cup raw cranberries (out of the freezer is fine) and a couple tablespoons of water. Explode the cranberries by cooking them in a saucepan with the water until they break down. Add 2 tsp Swerve or equivalent alternative natural sweetener, 1/2 tsp unflavored gelatin [optional] and 1/4 tsp cinnamon. Add a little orange zest if you're feeling fancy. Now you've got turkey with cranberry sauce. This sauce would go well with chicken, pork and veal, too.

Cranberries have about 12 g carbs per 100 g, so use them to create flavor, like this relish with your turkey, rather than as a full side dish. Especially with the combination of orange zest and cinnamon, the cranberry relish will taste really good; you should be able to use it sparingly and still get a lot of flavor. If you find it's hard to eat just a little, set it in the freezer until you're on Phase 3 of the diet. If eating just a little of something you enjoy is difficult, you may find the section called "A Taste of Honey" helpful.

Even after you've removed the skin, rotisserie chicken and turkey breast that were *cooked in their skin* at the grocery store will have higher fat than poultry with skin removed before cooking. Still, as a quick meal when you're too pooped to cook, rotisserie chicken or turkey breast with the skin removed is a fine choice on P2.

Whole turkey drumstick

Yes, you can have some dark meat! If you refer back to "Suggested Protein Choices" in this book, you'll see that a turkey leg is listed. Its protein density score is 7.8, as opposed to 19 for white meat turkey. You could eat a lot more turkey breast than turkey leg, but you might like the variety. Still, in terms of a quick bite that adds variety and packs to-go, it's nice to keep turkey legs in mind. Their protein density is a better choice for HCG is than trout, scallops and quite a few other items on the suggested proteins list.

Belgian endive with tuna salad

Endive makes great finger food. The leaves are sturdy enough to cradle things and they are tidy. **Tuna salad in endive leaves** looks just like an appetizer. A whole endive, sliced in half lengthwise, is also sturdy enough to put on the grill.

Sushi rolls

Dried seaweed (nori) sheets are sold in full and half sheets and a full sheet is only 10 calories. Many people miss sandwiches and wraps when on HCG and nori sheets are a clever ingredient. Make yourself a sushi-type roll (minus the rice) with traditional sushi roll ingredients such as **fresh crab and cucumber with wasabi.** Try also the combination of **raw tuna, shitake mushroom and pickled ginger.**

The best thing about sushi rolls as a quick snack, though, is that they put your leftovers to work for you. Try something unconventional, like **leftover meatball + kim chee + "honey mustard" in a nori wrap.**

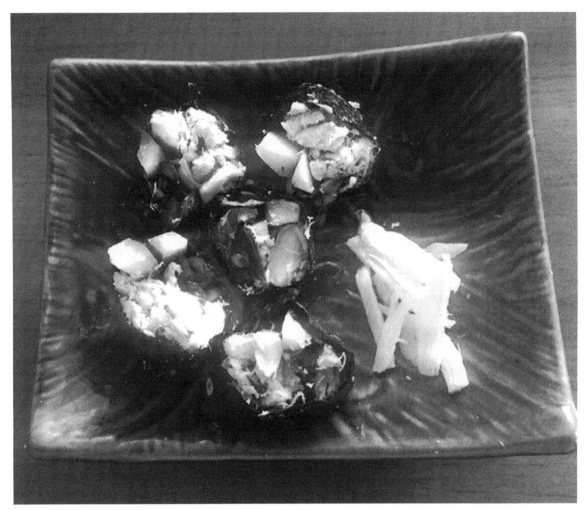

Photo: Dana Falk

Sushi rolls without rice present a physics challenge — they don't hold together terribly well — but fresh crab, marinated cucumber and radicchio with wasabi and pickled ginger are worth a little mess. HCG-friendly sushi rolls are something you could eat a lot of, too.

Turkey-pickle roll-ups

Remember that you can always use sliced meat as the *outside* of a wrap. This is messier to eat that a roll made with nori is, but it's a nice, filling snack. There's not much mystery to the ingredients that comprise a turkey-pickle roll-up, but for those who've had a hard day: a fresh pickle spear + condiment of choice ("honey" mustard, herbed cottage cheese, red pepper sauce, chopped kim chee, etc.) + slice of turkey wrapped around it.

Buying luncheon meat is tricky on HCG, because manufacturers may add dextrose, potato starch or tapioca starch. If your turkey slices have zero or < 1 carb per serving, you've found something safe for P2. (An item described < 1 carb on the nutritional information generally means that it has between .5 g and .95 g carbohydrate per serving. If it has less than .5 carbs per serving, manufacturers are allowed to list to as zero.) If the turkey luncheon meat in question has more than one carb, it probably contains starch of some kind.

Fresh pickles generally do not have added sugar. Brands like **Bubbies, Ba-Tempte, Grillo, Clausen, Sonoma Brinery, Britt's Pickles** and others makes fresh pickles that are kept in the refrigerated section at the grocery store, not on the shelf with the relishes and sweet pickles. The same goes for **sauerkraut**, though there are some sugar-free jars of sauerkraut and pickles that are shelf-stable. Any crisp pickle would be nice in your turkey roll-up. Of course if you've made your own refrigerator pickles, you're ahead of the game. Lots of ideas for aromatics (pickle flavorings) in the later section called "Refrigerator Pickles."

As for the condiments in your turkey-pickle roll-up, the majority of mustards are safe unless they say sweet-hot, maple mustard, honey mustard, etc. **Jalapeño mustard** usually has no sugar and it makes a great honey mustard once you've added a few drops of stevia glycerite to it. This "honey mustard" then forms the base of a salad dressing, a dip for leftover pork tenderloin or an even ingredient *inside* your meatloaf.

Whey Protein and Collagen Shakes

Whey protein isolate powder and bone broth protein powder can both be made into shakes that are quite filling. Choice of brand is important here, since some protein powders have sugar or use soy, rice, hemp or pea protein; these would be far less good for P2. **Thorne** makes high quality whey protein isolate; the vanilla flavor has 3 carbs per serving. **IsoPure** makes a zero carb whey powder in a number of good flavors, though these have a little sucralose, so don't rely heavily upon them.

If you are sensitive to dairy, *Ancient Nutrition* makes vanilla bone broth protein powder; it has 2 carbs, which is fine. There's also **goat whey protein powder** on the market for those who don't tolerate cow dairy. Some people love it and think it tastes swell, others think it tastes like the inside of a goat. Whatever your position, because whey protein does such an excellent job of making you feel full, it's worth looking into.

Why can't you buy just any protein powder? Because the amino acid profile of the protein source is what determines how your body will process it. Whey protein has the most robust amino acid profile, including essential branch chain amino acids. It has the capacity to satisfy hunger and support lean muscle mass much better than vegan protein sources do.

Look for a **hydrolyzed whey protein *isolate***; this means that the protein has been partially broken down and will be easier to digest. Lesser protein powders are more difficult to digest because they contain fillers in addition to the protein. Better not to risk that while on HCG.

See what kind of desserts you can concoct with whey protein isolate, but keep an eye on whether they cause cravings for you. To make a **protein powder mug cake,** mix a scoop (usually about 30 g) of whey protein powder (vanilla, chocolate, cookies and cream, cinnamon crunch, etc.) with an egg white and roughly 1.5 tbs water, tea or coffee,

DANA FALK, PH.D. & KELSEY KLAUSMEYER, N.D.

until you have something the consistency of pancake batter. Experiment with your ratio of liquid to protein powder to make the texture of mug cake you most enjoy.

Microwave your protein cake batter in a coffee mug, custard cup or small bowl/container for 45 seconds, then check it. It should look mostly done, with a little goo in the middle. (If a protein mug cake is fully cooked, especially with egg white but no yolk, it will be miserably, comically dense and chewy.) If the cake is not done, add just five seconds at a time in the microwave until cooked. If you prefer something fluffy and cake-like, err in the direction of undercooking it.

Try your finished product with a cup of coffee and see if it doesn't feel sorta-kinda like you're eating cake. On Phase 3, when you can eat egg yolks freely, that extra fat will produce a richer, more tender protein cake. These egg white only mug cakes are not luscious, but they can be satisfying. Feeling as though you've had dessert is likely to help you stop eating for the day.

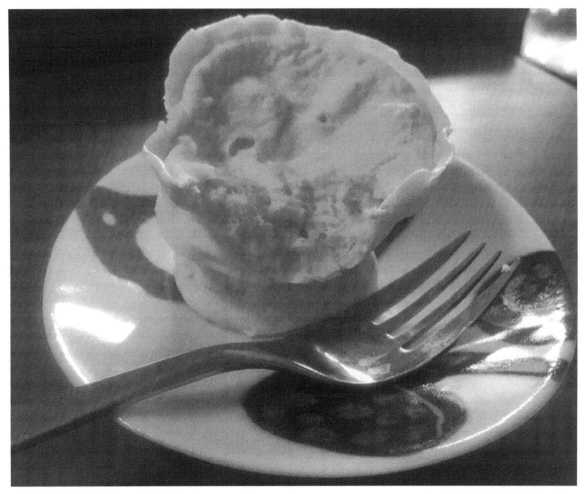

Photo: Dana Falk

This vanilla mug cake poses no threat to your neighborhood bakery, but it can hit the spot. This is Quest vanilla milkshake whey protein isolate + 1 large egg white + 1.5 tbs water in a custard cup. It is then microwaved 45 seconds. This one is a wee bit overdone as you can see — no goo in the center.

If you'd like to make **pumpkin mug cake,** use vanilla whey protein powder + two teaspoons of canned pumpkin + a dash of pumpkin pie spice or cinnamon + dash of salt. As long as you use **plain canned pumpkin** and not the sweetened "pumpkin pie filling," it's fine in small amounts on HCG. Canned pumpkin is on Tier 3, with exactly the same number of carbs per 100 g as fresh tomato.

Make a **whey protein shake** by crushing 12-15 ice cubes in your blender or food processor. Choose about 1/2 cup of a liquid: it may be water, coffee, chai tea, orange spice tea, etc. Add to the liquid a scoop of whey isolate protein powder to the crushed ice. From there, you can add flavor to the shake with cinnamon, turmeric powder, unsweetened cocoa powder, instant coffee, matcha green tea powder, natural flavor extracts, etc. For example, if you were to use **Quest cinnamon crunch whey protein powder** + chai tea you'd have a chai latte shake.

Think of a protein shake as a meal replacement if you're at the end of the day and almost out of calories. Nutritionally, it's not ideal, since substituting a protein shake for a meal means you're not getting diverse, whole foods. You will be more prone to nutrient and phytonutrient deficiencies if you rely too heavily upon protein shakes for your calories over a month or more of being on HCG. Because they help so much with satiety, try half a whey protein shake if you are very hungry before bed. Just half a shake (about 50 calories) might take the edge off your hunger and help you get to sleep more quickly.

Collagen powder

Collagen peptide powder is a safe, dairy-free alternative to whey protein. It's not as filling as whey protein is, but collagen offers the added benefit of supporting joints, skin, hair and nails, all of which may suffer on a low calorie diet.

If you cannot tolerate whey, collagen or bone broth protein, only then should you consider a vegan protein alternative. A rice/pea protein blend is a passable alternative, but you'd need to remain conscious of carb count, which varies greatly by brand.

Iced Teas

It's a little weird how satisfying a glass of iced tea is as compared with a glass of water. Buy yourself some unusual teas and keep a jug of iced tea in the fridge at all times while you're on HCG.

Orange or grapefruit rinds can soak in your jug of iced tea to impart that nice bitter essence without the carbs of eating an orange or grapefruit. **Chai or cinnamon spice tea infused with orange rind** is especially nice. **Black currant tea** is delicious iced. **Green tea with cucumber and/or fresh mint** infusing in the pitcher makes a light, refreshing iced tea.

High-quality flavor extracts help elevate iced tea. Ever paid $5 for lychee iced tea at a Thai restaurant? Make your own, with **unsweetened lychee extract.** A lot of people use flavored stevia drops, such as Sweet Leaf berry flavor, to make iced tea while on HCG. With good quality tea in your corner, you may not even need to sweeten it.

Here are a few specific suggestions for tea leaves you might consider:

Dried Hibiscus (*Jamaica* in Latino markets) makes a deep red tea, floral and slightly sour. Great infused with a cinnamon stick. Make extra for dessert ideas, below.

If you miss whiskey or beer, **Lapsang souchong tea and Assam tea** are both known for tasting malty. (In fact, they are too smoky and malty for some Western palates.) Try drinking in a highball glass on the rocks, if you think this would help. **Infusing malty teas overnight** with strong herbs like rosemary or sage will give them even more complexity, like a whisky. Of course it's not precisely like a cocktail, but creativity works in your favor.

Chrysanthemum tea is light and elegant. It's so floral it tastes slightly sweet. You can buy a big bag of dried chrysanthemum flowers at an Asian market rather inexpensively. Steep the chrysanthemum flowers for a long time, because the flavor is quite subtle. The flowers unfurl in the teapot, so it's a show-stopper.

Ginger peach iced tea is always a winner. It comes in decaf and is very good as an iced tea, especially if you've allowed fresh ginger to sit in it overnight and given it a few drops of **peach flavor extract.** (This is great iced tea when you're *not* on HCG, too.) Save some extra ginger peach tea for making gelatin squares or smoothies.

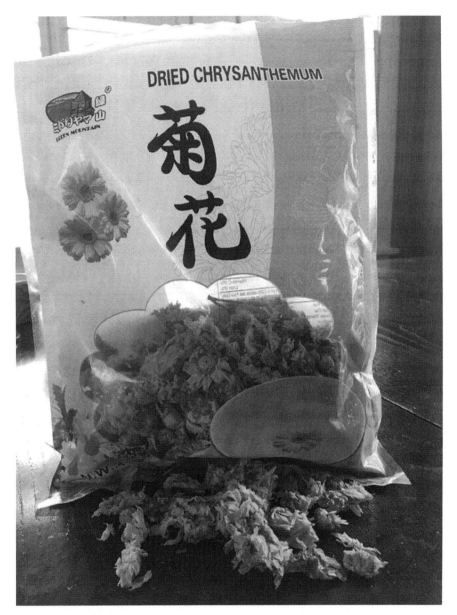

Photo: Dana Falk

Finding teas and coffees you enjoy is so useful for Phase 2. Chrysanthemum tea is very floral of course and can be a very nice way to wind down the day. It's light and delicate.

Carbonated Beverages Multi-Task!

Whether you call it soda water, seltzer, club soda, sparkling water, bubbly water, mineral water with gas or the utilitarian carbonated water, you've got something that's useful for your time on HCG.

(1) Soda water is quite filling. You can use it to help you feel fuller if you're still a little hungry at the end of a meal.

(2) You're supposed to drink a lot of water when trying to lose weight and plain soda water counts.

(3) Soda water is so plain, it takes on whatever flavor you give it: **flavored stevia drops, Ultima Replenishers electrolyte powder, fresh cucumber, fresh mint, fresh ginger, one smooshed strawberry** — you name it.

(4) When you make gelatin squares, you can replace some of the boiling water in the recipe with soda water.

(5) There are an increasing number of **seltzers that have fruit *essence*, but no sugar.** Treat yourself to an obscene variety of flavors and discover your favorites.

La Croix's mango seltzer is excellent. Their coconut seltzer with vanilla creme Sweet Leaf stevia drops makes an **HCG-friendly cream soda.** Target's house brand seltzer, **Simply Balanced**, tastes good and looks cool in tall, thin cans. (Is it superficial to admit a preference for the fun cans?) Kroger's house brand, **Simple Truth,** makes organic seltzer water in even cooler, taller cans with impressive flavor combinations like Tangerine Lemongrass, Mango Grapefruit, Cucumber Melon, Strawberry Watermelon, Blackberry Hibiscus and Orange Vanilla. There are many brands of flavored seltzer other than these on the market, so many flavors for you to try.

Fruit essence still water

If you prefer still water to carbonated, you'll probably love both **Hint Water** and **Ayala Herbal Water**. Both brands have flavor essence with no sweetener and both come in an impressive variety of flavors.

Hint waters are neither sweet nor sour; the flavors taste light and fresh. Particularly refreshing flavors are watermelon, blackberry and peppermint, in our humble opinion, with an honorable mention for lemon. The lemon does not taste sour as it would if you squeezed lemon juice into your water. Rather, it just has a light, fresh character. Hint's clementine flavor is lovely — mellow and soft, like ambrosia, rather than crisp.

Some brick and mortar stores carry Hint, but not in all of their flavors. Target and Walmart carry some Hint flavors, for example. Hint has variety packs that may help you locate your favorites (but not all of their flavors are included in those variety packs). Go to drinkhint.com for the complete selection of flavors.

Ayala Herbal Water comes in some lovely, unusual flavors: Lavender mint, lemongrass mint vanilla, ginger lemon peel and cinnamon orange peel, for example.

It may seem indulgent to pay for water in individual bottles — you certainly could fill your own water bottle and add some mint leaves — but it's a nice healthy treat for P2. Since drinking more water assists with weight loss, it seems a reasonable expense.

Both the seltzers and still waters with fruit *essence* are better for P2 than drinks sweetened with erythritol are, even though the latter do work for HCG. We suggest you save **Bai drinks, Everly drink mixes, Zevia soda, Dry Soda Zero Sugar, Ultima Replenishers** (and other drinks with alternative natural sweeteners) for making treats like **popsicles, granitas and gelatin desserts**. For drinking as much water as possible, focus on the flavor essence waters and sodas mentioned in this section.

Refrigerator Pickles

Refrigerator pickles are the HCG quick bite that has earned its own section. Pickles work hard on your behalf because you can chop them to make a **relish,** slice them thinly to create a crisp **side dish,** add pickled veggies to your **meat roll-up or nori wraps** or make **whole, gourmet pickles** to bring on a picnic. Our patients say that they miss *flavor* when they're on Phase 2 and tangy pickled vegetables may be a help.

Refrigerator pickles are a blast to make if you enjoy playing with flavor, because you begin with a basic brine and use aromatics to build the flavor profile you enjoy. These pickles are not fermented, just refrigerated in homemade brine, so are ready to eat in three hours.

Veggies you could pickle

Good heavens, don't limit yourself to cucumbers. Any HCG-friendly veggie that is sturdy has pickling potential:

Raw or blanched cauliflower
Raw or blanched green beans
Radishes
Pickling cucumbers or Persian cucumbers
Blanched asparagus
Celery
Cabbage

Kohlrabi
Green tomatoes
Bell peppers
Fresh fennel bulb
Mustard greens or turnip greens
Jalapeños
Brussels sprouts

Your leftover glass jars will work perfectly well, as long as they have a wide mouth and a tight-fitting lid. Put them through a hot dishwasher cycle to clean them. This is not the level of sterilization one needs when preserving food and expecting it to be safe to eat in a year. Refrigerator pickles are not fermented, so they only last a couple weeks in the fridge. You simply need very clean jars and lids that have been washed in very hot water.

Let's begin with a boilerplate recipe for refrigerator pickles, then move to some ideas for how you might personalize the flavors.

Basic Refrigerator Pickle Recipe

This makes one quart of pickles. Consider splitting the recipe to make two pints of pickles that are different, rather than a whole quart with a single flavor profile.

Materials

One quart-size or two pint-size glass jars with lids

Pickling veggies

1 pound (16 oz) vegetable of choice (or 8 oz each of two veggies)

Brine

1/2 cup water

1 1/2 cups unsweetened apple cider vinegar, rice vinegar or coconut vinegar

Whole, dry spice(s) of choice: allspice, celery seeds, fennel seeds, mustard seeds, tea leaves, peppercorns, coriander, star anise, etc.

1-inch cube of fresh ginger or 1 large garlic clove, peeled and halved. Using both is fine.

Fresh herb(s) of choice: mint, basil, tarragon, lemongrass, thyme, dill, fennel fronds, marjoram, sage, chives, oregano. If you want something that will fade into the background, try basil, marjoram, jasmine tea or fennel fronds.

2 tsp granular Swerve or 7 drops Stevia glycerite

Note: *This is the amount of sweetener you'd use for savory pickles, not sweet ones.* Two teaspoons is just enough sweetness to give the brine some balance if you're making kosher dills, for example, or pickles that are intended to be spicy, earthy or herbaceous. You will add much more sweetener if you're aiming for something sweet and sour, like the Thai sweet n' spicy pickles or the curried bread and butter pickles, listed below.

1. Thoroughly wash jar(s) in hot water or run through dishwasher.

2. Combine all brine ingredients, except the fresh herbs, in a saucepan. Heat to a low boil, stir to incorporate then remove from heat.

3. While brine is heating, wash and trim the veggies you plan to pickle. Cut to desired size.

4. Place fresh herb(s) in the bottom of each clean jar.

5. Fill jar most of the way with veggies, packing them loosely enough for brine to circulate.

6. Once brine is warm but not hot, pour it to cover veggies in jars.

7. Let jars sit on counter, uncovered, until at room temperature.

8. Once cooled, place lids tightly on jars and refrigerate.

Pickles should be ready to eat in three hours. If after three hours they don't taste like much, add pungent aromatics like raw garlic, fresh ginger or fresh jalapeños, add more vinegar or a powerful dry spice like star anise or Sichuan peppercorns. If they are too tart from the vinegar after three hours, dilute with water.

Pickling Flavor Combinations

The recipe above is for a generic pickling brine. It's very good, but will be better if you swap-in the flavors you most enjoy. Here are some flavor combinations to inspire your artisan pickling career:

... Cloves, stevia and one Thai chile = **sweet and sour pickle with a little heat**

... Dill, allspice, celery seed, peppercorns and mustard seed = **traditional deli pickle**

... Fresh ginger, lemon, lime or grapefruit slices + fresh mint = **clean, refreshing pickle**

... Fresh garlic and jalapeños = **savory and spicy pickle**

... Fresh turmeric and orange slices = **earthy flavor, bright orange color**

... Lime, kaffir lime leaves, lemongrass = **subtle Thai herb pickle**

... Curry powder, sweetener, allspice, fennel = **curried sweet pickle**

Aromatics by flavor profile

If you prefer, create a signature refrigerator pickle recipe from square one. Choose whatever aromatics will combine to make the pickles you most enjoy:

✒ Sour

Lemon, lime

Grapefruit, pomelo

Kumquat

Vinegars: apple cider, rice, coconut, white wine, tarragon

Dried hibiscus flowers

Rhubarb

Sour cherries

Green papaya

Green mango

✒ Hot

Fresh Thai chiles, habanero, scotch bonnet

Jalapeños, Anaheim, pasilla peppers

Peppercorns

Galanga (young ginger)

Horseradish root

Wasabi root

✒ Spicy or pungent, but not hot

Turmeric root

Ginger root

Cardamom pods

Cumin seeds

Mustard seeds

Saffron

Whole cloves

Whole allspice

Star anise

Curry powder

Garlic cloves

Chives

❧ Herbaceous

Fresh mint

Fresh dill

Fresh thyme or rosemary

Fresh basil or tarragon

Lemongrass

Marjoram

Celery root, stalks or leaves

Caraway seeds

Fennel bulb, fronds or seeds

❧ Sweet

Alternative natural sweeteners

Vanilla bean

Large pieces of fruit (for flavor only)

Rose water

Orange blossom water
Whole cinnamon sticks

❧ Bitter

Citrus peel (especially grapefruit, pomelo)
Juniper berries
Green tea leaves
Bay leaves
Kaffir lime leaves

❧ Briny

Lavender salt
Rosemary salt
Smoked cherrywood or applewood salt
Smoked maldon salt
Clam juice
Fresh oysters

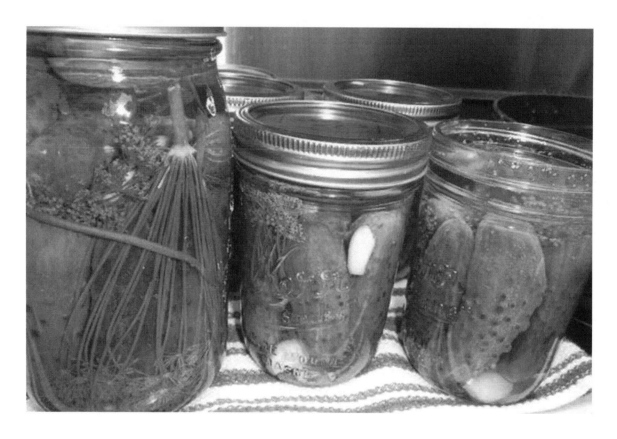

The aromatics you choose make all the difference for refrigerator pickles. A few cloves of garlic and your favorite fresh herbs create a pickle that's tasty and unique. Spicy pickles, curried pickles and sweet relish can all be yours.

Homemade Jerky

If you have a food dehydrator, you've got the potential to make all kinds of treats for yourself while on the HCG Diet. You can make **dried vegetables like crunchy green beans, chewy dried fruit like sour starfruit slices and dried meats like bison or turkey jerky.** There are entire cookbooks devoted to what can be made in a dehydrator — from homemade yogurt to dehydrated onion dip mix to liver dog treats — but we focus here only on homemade jerky because it's filling, shelf stable and travels well.

A food dehydrator is not absolutely essential to making jerky, but it's more reliable than using your oven at low temperature is. It's also less worrisome because it turns itself off. Food dehydrators are notorious counter space hogs, but they're a neat toy that would be useful long after HCG, so consider it.

Full-sized food dehydrators can accommodate about 45 pieces of jerky. When dried, the meat shrinks in size and weight such that three pounds of meat makes about one pound of finished jerky.

What follows is a boilerplate recipe for teriyaki-style jerky and a list of flavor ideas to inspire your own creations. The marinade is the key to what your jerky will taste like, of course, but there are other factors at play, too: which meat you use, how thinly you slice it and how long you marinate it. For example, bland turkey meat would be overwhelmed by a salty marinade much more quickly than richer bison meat would be.

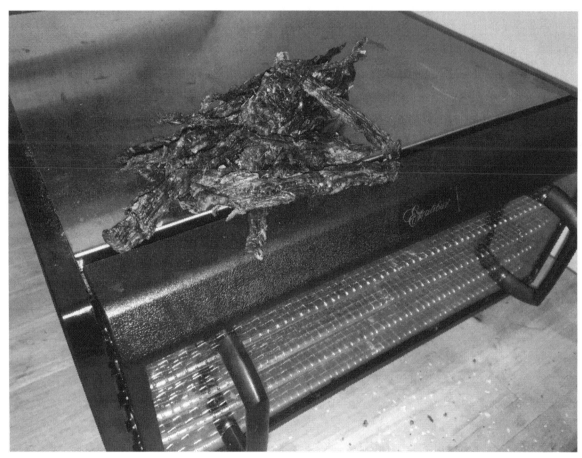

Photo: Dana Falk

This pile of beef jerky (18-20 small pieces) was made from drying one pound of top round beef for nine hours at 165° F. You may decide to marinate several pounds of meat at a time, to produce a larger batch of jerky. Pop into a zipper bag and your jerky is shelf stable for several weeks at least.

Basic Teriyaki Jerky Marinade

This teriyaki-style marinade goes well with most meats — red meat like bison or beef, a slightly sweet meat like pork or goat. To use it with a more delicate protein like cod or turkey, you'll reduce the amount of time it's in the marinade.

TIP: The bottom line with any teriyaki is that it's sweet and salty. If you don't have the energy for making the gourmet teriyaki marinade that appears here, just toss some sliced, very lean meat into a zipper bag, with coconut aminos and a few pinches of salt for an hour. The meat will turn out sorta-kinda like teriyaki jerky.

On P2, all your proteins must be super lean, so be prepared for a tough and chewy finished product. Dense homemade jerky will still be a welcome snack on HCG, but keep hope alive — your jerky after HCG will be far more luscious. You will eventually be able to dehydrate flank steak for a more tender beef jerky or salmon for a richer flavor, for example.

You'll also have a wider variety of fruits and vegetables to dehydrate after HCG. Sliced kiwis, for example, turn out chewy, sweet and sour when they've been dried in a food dehydrator; they make a beautiful, bright green gift for someone.

For now, let's work on making some delightfully tough teriyaki jerky.

Teriyaki Jerky

Marinates up to 1.5 pounds of meat
Combine ingredients in a zipper bag, glass pan or plastic container

1 cup coconut aminos
2 1/2 tbs tamari
3 tbs apple cider vinegar, rice vinegar or coconut vinegar
Ideal sweetener: 3 tbs. Sukrin Gold or Swerve Brown (it's like brown sugar)
Alternative: Up to 1/2 tsp stevia glycerite (not regular stevia drops)
2 tsp chopped fresh ginger (more if you love it)
1.5 tsp fresh lime juice
Dash cinnamon [up to 1/8 tsp]
Dash onion powder [up to 1/8 tsp]

Optional additions:

Hot sauce or hot chilis
1 tsp chopped fresh garlic [more if you love it]
Pineapple or mango flavor extract [not juice]
Orange zest
2+ tbs All-u-Lose or Choc Zero maple syrup
Dash ground clove [an excellent addition]
Whole allspice, whole cinnamon stick

Combine all marinade ingredients and adjust for the balance of salty/sweet/spicy/sour you like. You may leave any citrus seeds, ginger peels, chili tops and such in the marinade.

Slice meat to about 1/4 inch thickness. Pound slices to all be roughly the same thickness.

Add sliced, pounded meat to marinade in bowl, pan or bag. Refrigerate 3-4 hours. Halfway through the marinating process, rotate bottom slices to top, so all are getting the marinade.

Drain marinated meat and pat dry *thoroughly*. Remove as much moisture as possible.

Place meat slices in food dehydrator, allowing as much space between pieces as possible.

Set dehydrator temperature to 160° F to 165° F degrees. Set timer for 9 hours. Drying time will depend upon how thickly the meat is sliced.

The jerky is done when it has no visible moisture from fat or marinade. It should still be pliable (chewy), not yet brittle.

Start checking the jerky at 8 hours. If you had any small pieces they may already be done. The rest should be done by 9 hours.

Store finished jerky in a zipper bag or airtight container.

Engineering Flavor Combinations

There are many ways to be inventive with cooking, even during HCG Phase 2, but each of us has only so many ideas. Not only that, some flavors go well together, but they're not combinations we personally have experienced, so we'd never think to try them.

If you believe that maximizing flavor and being inventive while on HCG will help you to succeed, there's a terrific resource you should be aware of. There's a book called *The Flavor Bible* by Karen Page and Andrew Dornenburg (2008). This book enables you to search for an ingredient of interest and see what flavors professional chefs say go well with it. *The Flavor Bible* can thus help you to engineer new recipes while on P2. The text is available as a physical book and as an electronic book.

Let's play with our own example of engineering a flavor combination specific to HCG. Pork tenderloin is a protein you can eat on HCG Phase 2. Below are all the ingredients we can think of that you might pair with pork tenderloin. (So as not to be cruel, we're only mentioning flavors you could use while on Phase 2.)

Pork Tenderloin

Goes well with: adobo sauce, allspice, anise, arugula, basil, cabbage, caraway, cardamom, cauliflower, celeriac, celery, chai tea, chanterelle mushrooms, Chinese bitter melon (*foo gwa* or *fu gua*), chrysanthemum, cinnamon, coconut vinegar, cranberry, curry, fennel, fenugreek, galanga, garlic, ginger, green tabasco, green tea, horseradish, kumquat, lavender, lavender salt, lemon thyme, lemon verbena, lemongrass, marjoram, pickled onions, radicchio, rhubarb, rosemary, saffron, sage, sauerkraut, Sichuan peppercorn, star anise, sweet peppers, tarragon, wasabi, white pepper.

The more difficult repetition is for you, the more helpful it will be to expand your repertoire in this way, engineering unique flavor in your cooking. If you'd like to delve more into the connection between your personality traits and your strategy for the HCG Diet, be sure to read the section "Personal Insights Useful for Weight Loss" that comes later in the book.

Tricks with Alternative Natural Sweeteners

You can also engineer flavor while on HCG with the help of safe sweeteners. Adding just a touch of sweetness can make a big difference to a wide variety of dishes and condiments, so the ideas here are certainly not limited to desserts. For example, creating a slightly sweet stir-fry sauce may make your savory dishes more satisfying.

If you need a refresher on the sweeteners we refer to in this chapter, hop back to the section "Alternative Natural Sweeteners." There are a large number of choices and some people have a real preference for liquid, like Better Stevia, or powdered, like Swerve Confectioner's.

Here are some things you can create with a touch of an alternative natural sweetener like stevia glycerite, monk fruit extract, allulose, erythritol or xylitol:

1. Vinegar or lemon juice + sweetener = sweet and sour flavor

Citrus juice + MCT oil + mustard + a little sweetener = a pretty darn good **vinaigrette for chicken salad, tuna salad, cole slaw, calamari salad** and such. Vinegar is lower in calories than citrus juice is and it has no carbs, so use it when you can, but some dishes really benefit from that citrus flavor. A **chilled calamari salad** would be awesome with some lemon juice in the vinaigrette, for example.

If you add fresh ginger and citrus zest to the above vinaigrette, it's a **marinade for fresh halibut, ahi tuna steak or pork tenderloin.** Omit the MCT oil if you're using it for a marinade that will later be cooked, since MCT oil has an extremely low smoke point.

Strained tomato + cider vinegar + fish sauce + sweetener + salt + ground cinnamon, clove and allspice + xanthan gum (optional) = **sweet and sour sauce.**

Sweet and sour sauce looks like a lot of ingredients, but it's worth the effort. Cook it down in a saucepan to thicken. This is tomato-based, so use it sparingly, but sweet and sour sauce really perks up a dry protein.

2. Mustard + liquid sweetener = honey mustard

Honey mustard works as a **dip for leftover meatballs, a condiment for making lettuce wraps, an accompaniment to a pork tenderloin and sauerkraut dinner, the base of a dressing for a cold salad or a hot vegetable.** Honey mustard is quite handy to have around on P2.

Most supermarket mustard does not have sugar, unless it's called maple mustard, sweet-hot mustard, cranberry mustard or honey mustard, but read the label to be certain. An ingredient tip: **Choc Zero** and **All-u-lose** are brands that make delicious syrups, like honey, vanilla, peach, caramel, maple and maple-pecan. These would be great for creating "honey mustard" if used in small amounts. Both brands use alternative natural sweeteners: Choc Zero uses monk fruit extract and All-u-lose uses allulose.

3. Strained tomato + vinegar + sweetener + salt + onion powder = ketchup

Plain ketchup is very useful, and with just a few more ingredients, you have interesting variations. Add curry powder for a **German curry ketchup**, hot sauce for a **spicy ketchup,** crushed celery seed or fennel seed for **marinara sauce,** horseradish for

cocktail sauce. Reduce your ingredients in a saucepan to get a more concentrated flavor and thicker consistency.

Refrigerate some of your ketchup and freeze the rest in an ice cube tray. An egg white with spinach for breakfast is less depressing with a bit of homemade ketchup.

4. Tamari + sweetener = teriyaki

Note: There's a tastier, more gourmet recipe for teriyaki sauce in the section "Homemade Jerky." The suggestion here is just a simple hack using sweetener.

If you want the consistency of a thick **teriyaki sauce**, make your sweetener **Sukrin fiber syrup or Choc Zero maple syrup.** These have a thick consistency like corn syrup but are not sugars or artificial sweeteners; they are alternative natural sweeteners just like stevia is. Sukrin and Choc Zero products are generally purchased online, so order this as soon as you think you may need it. Another way to thicken any sauce is to add a tiny pinch of xanthan gum and simmer it until it reduces.

If you'd like a thinner teriyaki marinade for meat or seafood that you will grill later, your sweetener can be any alternative natural sweetener you wish: liquid, granular, powdered or a brown sugar substitute like **Swerve Brown and Sukrin Gold.** The brown sugar substitutes would make your sauce taste the most like real teriyaki.

Likewise, if your plan is to soak shirataki noodles in your teriyaki marinade before sautéing them, you may use any alternative natural sweetener you would like. **Shirataki noodles** take some time to absorb the flavor you're giving them, so allow an hour or so in the teriyaki marinade. Once marinated, **teriyaki noodles sautéed with shredded cabbage** makes a filling, substantial side dish for nearly no calories.

5. Hot coffee or chai tea + MCT oil + cinnamon + sweetener = cappuccino or creamy chai

If you combine extra strong coffee or chai spice tea with some alternative natural sweetener, a dash of cinnamon and 1 tablespoon of MCT oil, then put it in the blender, it becomes a **creamy chai or cappuccino.**

TIP: Your hot, creamy beverage will quickly drop in temperature when it's whipped in the blender. If this matters to you, begin by making your coffee or tea extra hot, in the microwave, then blend your drink just long enough to make it frothy.

Some patients tell us that they save some of their MCT oil and sweetener specifically for an evening beverage; that's a great idea. Creating a routine that includes a creamy, sweet drink for dessert each night associates that cappuccino or chai with the end of your eating for the day. Any practice that you use to mark the end of eating prevents late night snacking.

6. Unflavored gelatin + safe fruit drinks = gelatin dessert

It's easy to make a gelatin dessert that keeps you away from more caloric choices. Unflavored gelatin may be purchased in bags and canisters, not just in little packets and it's a good investment.

Everly powdered drink mixes are made with erythritol. They are very concentrated powders that come in pomegranate-berry, mango-peach, strawberry-lemonade and fruit punch, for example.

Ultima Replenisher electrolyte drink mixes are made with stevia. If all these virtuous recipes for baked fish make you feel like having a drink that's electric blue, Ultima makes a delightful **blue raspberry flavor** that may scratch that itch.

Bai drinks are already mixed and bottled. They come in a huge variety of flavors and are sweetened with stevia and erythritol combined. Bai sells variety packs, so you can try a number of flavors at once, if you wish. Coconut pineapple is fabulous, as is peach, blueberry lemonade and mango...there's not a bad one in the bunch, actually. An easy, satisfying Phase 2 recipe would be to make **gelatin dessert squares** using an 18-ounce bottle of Bai drink in any flavor you would like.

Gelatin Dessert Squares

You'll need a glass pan between 7 x 9 inches and 9 x 13 inches.

2.5 cups (20 oz) water + 2 tsp Everly drink powder, boiling hot
OR
1 bottle (18 oz) Bai drink + 2 oz water, boiling hot

3.5 tbs or 4 envelopes unflavored gelatin (more for gummies; see below)
1/8 tsp salt
Optional: 1/2 tsp citric acid powder for sweet and sour flavor

— Place the unflavored gelatin and salt in the glass pan. Add citric acid, if using.
Use 2.5 tbs gelatin if you want a dessert you eat with a spoon
Use 3.5 tbs gelatin if you like gelatin squares that are finger food (this recipe)
Use 5 tbs gelatin if you'd like chewy gelatin that's gummy bear consistency.

— Bring the drink to a full boil and pour into the pan. Whisk immediately, until the gelatin is completely incorporated.

— Leave hot gelatin in pan on the counter for 20 minutes, then refrigerate at least 90 min.

— Once solid, cut into squares and you've got a satisfying little dessert that's finger food.

The *entire pan* has 91 calories and one net carb. Cutting the gelatin dessert into squares makes it easy to visualize how much you've eaten.

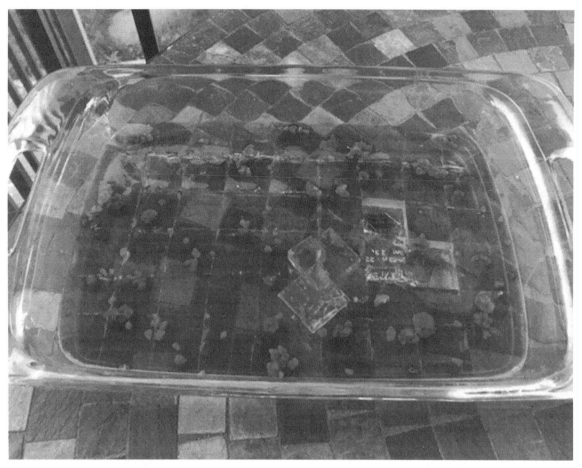

Photo: Dana Falk

These fun gelatin squares were made with Everly berry-pomegranate drink mix, 1/2 tsp citric acid and a few frozen raspberries. They taste like sweet and sour berry gummies and are easy to portion for yourself.

Your gelatin squares or gummies may be made of beverages other than fruit-flavored drinks, of course. You might try creating your own blends, like **green tea with a little pureed casaba melon. Also try ginger peach tea with freshly grated ginger or Choc Zero peach syrup.**

Since you'll want to minimize sweeteners, consider using Everly or Bai drinks as popsicles, gelatin desserts or granita rather than chugging them as drinks. If you drink them, consider diluting them beyond the recommended proportions. They only have five calories, so that's not the issue; it's that sweeteners can increase hunger. For example, **Ultima Replenisher Electrolyte drinks** recommend mixing one scoop or "stickpacket" with 2 cups of water. We think it tastes great in 3 1/2 cups water, though! The same is true for Everly drink mixes, which still taste very good when diluted more than is suggested on the package. Doing this would save you money, too.

TIP: Ultima makes several flavors, including a tasty orange drink that may remind you of *Tang*. Ultima orange makes a nice breakfast drink that stands-in for orange juice or a tasty orange granita (see below) that costs you zero calories.

7. Strong iced tea or other drink frozen into ice cubes + water + sweetener + blender = frozen dessert

If you remember to freeze some of your favorite drink in an ice cube tray, you'll be glad you did. Crush these flavorful ice cubes in the blender or food processor. This becomes a **sorbet** if you add a tiny bit of water, a **granita** if you add a medium amount of water and a **slushy drink** if you add a lot.

Experiment with flavor. Adding just a couple of **frozen raspberries or blackberries** brings a lot of flavor. Try **Everly strawberry-lemonade with a little frozen strawberry** in it. Try **Earl grey tea with a little lemon and vanilla.**

DANA FALK, PH.D. & KELSEY KLAUSMEYER, N.D.

This same process may be applied to the Bai drinks, of course. Bai makes a **coconut lime drink** that would be great as a slushy with just a squeeze of fresh lime juice.

308

Video, Recipe and Workbook Resources

If detailed recipes are more your style than cooking strategies are, remember that there are recipes for HCG Phases 2 and 3 on the internet, on YouTube and in published cookbooks. If you like structure more than improvisation, you may want to seek resources that put some organization in place for you.

Rayzel Lam has written an HCG workbook, produced a collection of YouTube videos about the diet, has created recipes, a website, a blog and a special program for maintenance beyond Phase 3. She goes by *HCG Chica* and her website is www.hcgchica.com.

We appreciate that the HCG Chica's contributions are more visual, more intimate and more concrete than ours are and we believe her offerings could be a valuable resource for our readers. She herself was highly successful on the diet and now assists others with information and inspiration.

Whether you're approaching the diet from an *HCG for Foodies* perspective or are following the original protocol faithfully, you're likely to find ***HCG Chica's HCG Diet Workbook*** very helpful. This workbook is different from our book, in a good way! For example, while we explain how HCG interacts metabolically with your food choices, the HCG Chica workbook is an interactive tool that enables you to track those daily choices. We think this combination of tools would be dynamite for your success on HCG.

We think *HCG for Foodies* and the *HCG Chica's HCG Diet Workbook* complement each other in a number of ways:

We explain...	...and the workbook helps with
How to design goals for HCG based on endocrinology and psychology...	...a way to track your progress on those goals
How to choose specific foods that work for you...	...a way to visually organize what you actually chose to eat each day
Detailed, active preparations for the diet...	...grocery lists and other tools you can print out as you prepare
Diverse strategies for changing an important behavior...	...an opportunity to take notes on your changes as you make them
Challenges HCG patients bring to the doctor's office and strategies that help them overcome these...	...support and vision from someone who overcame challenges herself and who gathers others' success stories
Personality insights like fear of weight loss, assertiveness, adaptability and need for freedom...	...confidence and resilience, such as how to fix a cheat or how to cope with a weight loss stall

HCG Chica's HCG Diet Workbook is also re-usable, particularly if you buy the digital version at her website. The digital workbook can be read on a tablet or phone, has printable worksheets and becomes interactive with your download of a free reader app. Her workbook enables you to do detailed daily tracking and journaling, has printable food lists, a troubleshooting log and lots of encouragement.

The **HCG Chica's YouTube videos** are also very valuable, in our opinion. These videos are a deep dive into the specifics of life on the diet. She shares her own journey, a very significant weight loss she has kept off for many years. She clarifies that she is not a healthcare professional but rather is addressing questions about the HCG diet from her experience. HCG Chica videos are a terrific resource not just for the information she shares but for the companionship they provide. This diet, especially on Phase 2, can feel a bit isolating.

On her website, the HCG Chica also offers **innovative recipes.** These are precise recipes with nutritional breakdown, as opposed to the cooking and flavor ideas we provide. Two sets of recipes are presented: one that uses only ingredients on the original Simeons protocol (Specific Protocol or SP) and a second set that includes additional ingredients (Alternate Protocol or AP). Ingredients are considered Alternate Protocol if weight loss clinics find their HCG patients still lose weight effectively while eating these foods.

Deserving of special mention are HCG Chica recipes for:

Egg drop soup
Vietnamese caramelized shrimp
Blended mushroom soup
Maple smoked chipotle chicken
Cottage pie with radish mash
Zucchini lasagne
Moroccan chicken stew
Cheesesteak stacks minus the cheese sauce

Finally, check out the ***HCG Chica's P3 to Life Maintenance Program.*** It's structured help with what to eat after HCG (or between rounds of it) when you want to maintain but aren't sure how to do that. Some of the HCG Chica's followers expressed interest in something more directive for life after the diet. What she created in response is just that. Specific foods and serving sizes. Meals plans and their corresponding recipes. Grocery lists. Video tutorials about shopping and cooking for the maintenance phase. Videos that coach you through the mental and emotional challenges. The *P3 to Life Maintenance Program* is not a book, it's a multi-media resource.

In all, we hope you'll avail yourself of these or any resources that you find complement *HCG for Foodies*.

Beware these ingredients in recipes online

There are some terrific ideas on the internet for HCG Phase 2 cooking, but not all recipes are equally reliable. Here are some ingredients we've noticed in online recipes that we have reservations about:

— Bean sprouts (estrogenic)
— Pears, apples, oranges, apricots (fructose)
— Peanut butter powder (carbs, fat)
— Better Than Bullion (sugar, corn syrup, food starch)
— Psyllium husk powder (rapid weight gain, carbs)
— Egg yolks (fat)

Chocolate soufflé mini cake

Now for some hypocrisy: here is *our* idea for a dessert with an ingredient that's strange for HCG Phase 2. We have found that making a tiny cake using unsweetened cocoa powder can be very helpful for addressing a lack of treats on P2. In fact, some patients say that this little microwave cake is what enabled them to remain on the very low calorie diet.

Several brands of unsweetened cocoa powder have only 10 calories, 1/2 gram of fat and 3 g total carbs / 1g net carbs per tablespoon. By comparison, 1/3 cup of fresh strawberries (on the original Simeons HCG protocol) has 15 calories, 3.6 g total carbs / 2.6 g net carbs.

So this recipe for chocolate soufflé mini cake is unconventional but it does make logical sense for ketosis. You'll notice that the high-end brands of unsweetened cocoa powder are generally no good for HCG because they have a higher fat content. However, **Hershey's 100% cacao (unsweetened) cocoa powder** does work, in both regular and Special Dark versions. This unsweetened cocoa has only 10 calories per tablespoon and that's an awful lot of flavor for a 10 calorie investment!

Again, our philosophy: if eating a little bit of something that tastes good is the difference between continuing the low calorie diet and giving up (or binging) have something tasty. Eating a large portion of an HCG-friendly food is far wiser than eating anything with sugar, fat or starch is. We think this chocolate soufflé mini-cake is a safe bet.

Chocolate Soufflé Mini-Cake

1 egg white
1 tbs MCT oil
12-15 drops *Better Stevia* glycerite or 1 tsp alternative natural sweetener

1 tbs unsweetened cocoa powder (any brand with .5 gram fat and 3 g carb, such as Hershey's)
1/4 tsp baking powder
Up to 1/8 tsp kosher salt

Recommended: 10 grams (about 1 tbs) peeled, raw zucchini, crookneck squash or summer squash. (The grated squash can't be tasted in the soufflé, it just gives you a larger cake to enjoy for nearly no additional calories.)

Optional: 1/8 - 1/4 tsp instant coffee

— Find a ramekin, custard cup, or other small container about 4 inches across.

— Whisk together the egg white, MCT oil, salt and sweetener.

— Add the grated zucchini (if using) and combine well.

— Add the dry ingredients: cocoa, baking powder + instant coffee and/or cinnamon, if using.

— Combine thoroughly, until ingredients come together as a smooth batter (this requires some effort).

— Microwave for one minute if you like a moist middle, like a lava cake, or 1 minute and 10 seconds if you want it drier, like a piece of cake.

— Enjoy your 31 calorie treat (29 cals without the zucchini.)

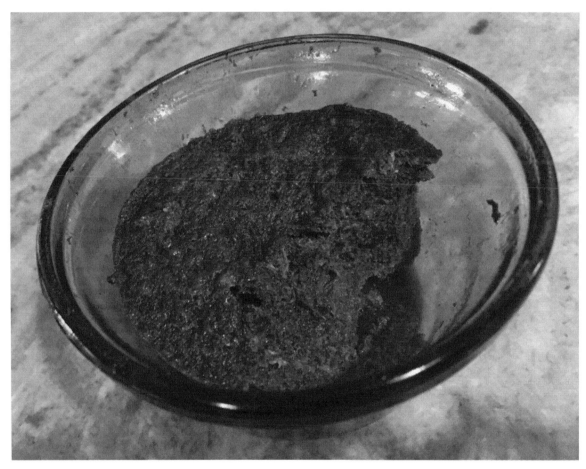

Photo: Dana Falk

This is the texture of a chocolate soufflé mini-cake that was microwaved for one minute, 10 seconds in a 4-inch wide custard cup. The larger the bowl you use, the less time your mini-cake will need to cook. If you want the cake to be gooey, begin by microwaving it for 50 seconds.

The Purpose of HCG Phase 3

Once you have lost weight on HCG Phase 2, your job is to guard this accomplishment like a junkyard dog. There's a specific method for managing this transition; we give you those specifics in this chapter.

You will gradually increase your calories and slowly re-introduce fats in Phase 3 (P3.) Plan to increase your diet 100-200 calories per day until you reach the target number of calories your healthcare provider has recommended. You'll then hold at this number of calories for about three weeks, which encourages your body to establish your new weight as your "set point."

Ask your healthcare provider for your personal target calories while on HCG Phase 3. Many practitioners set that target at 100 calories below your basal metabolic rate (BMR.) If you don't know your current basal metabolic rate, that information is worth seeking out. Getting a Bioelectrical Impedance Analysis (BIA) is one way to gather this information; these are often available at natural medicine clinics. Your primary care team may have another method for assessing your metabolic rate, though.

If you haven't had a caloric goal recommended for you, and you can't access your basal metabolic rate, try 1,200 calories a day as your initial goal.

For people who've had trouble losing weight or keeping it off, knowing your metabolic rate can be sort of a relief! People who have had endocrine or digestive system issues, who have a family tendency towards higher body mass index or who are in menopause sometimes say that if they learn their metabolism actually *is* low, it's encouraging. They now have evidence that they really do gain weight more easily than the average person does.

On the flip side, if your metabolic rate is perfectly normal, it may mean that you have had difficulty losing weight or keeping it off because you lacked information about how to do that. Now that research shows how eating low fat is not the most effective way to lose weight, this may be a happy time for you. You might choose to embark on a low carbohydrate (ketogenic) diet, starting with HCG. Low carbohydrate diets are generally easier to sustain than low fat diets are.

The goal on HCG Phase 3 is to stabilize within several pounds of your last "dose weight," which is your weight on the last day you took a shot, sub-lingual tablet or drops of HCG. Your target calories during P3 are lower than after you're done with the diet, so don't worry. The goal is not for you to eat 100 calories below your metabolic rate forever, it's just a strategy to help you stick the landing after all your hard work on Phase 2.

Important: Your absolute lowest weight will probably be a few days after your final dose of HCG. This is water loss, so *don't make this the weight you're trying to stabilize!* Your scale weight on the last day you took the hormone is what's relevant.

The purpose of HCG Phase 3 is not to freak you out about food for life. Once your weight has stabilized, we hope you will diversify your diet. Our patients sometimes get fixated on the restrictive aspect of HCG — all the things they have to rule *out* — and they forget to bring foods back into the rotation after they're done with HCG. Your gut microbiome needs a variety of phytonutrients from a variety of foods. Since metabolism is one of the functions your microbiome handles, having a more diverse diet is a good long-term goal.

Days immediately following Phase 2

The original Simeons protocol directs patients to continue eating 500 calories for three full days after their final dose of the hormone. That's awfully tough to do. For most people, the HCG has been fully metabolized and has moved through their body after just 24 hours. How quickly your particular liver would metabolize the hormone is not data we have easy access to.

Here's the practical way to know when it's safe to start increasing your caloric intake: once you feel ravenously hungry eating only 500-800 calories. Once that happens, we know the HCG has moved through you. *For the first 24 hours after your final dose of HCG, absolutely stick to the low calorie diet.* There's no question about that. From there on, we suggest you compare how hungry you felt when on the hormone to how hungry you feel now. When you are ridiculously hungry on very low calories, it's safe to start increasing calories, even if it's been less than three days time.

Once natural hunger returns, the HCG has passed through you and it's safe to begin adding 100-200 calories per day. For a few people, it will take the full three days noted in the original protocol, but do consider moving on to Phase 3 once you feel natural hunger return. The longer you eat very few calories, the greater the risk your basal metabolic rate will go down.

If you don't care for guesswork, do this: remain on the very low calorie diet, without the hormone, for two full days.

Successful pacing on P3

The key to HCG Phase 3 is "slow and steady wins the race." Being exquisitely patient about returning fat and calories to your diet will have five important benefits for you:

1. *It preserves your metabolism, thus your weight loss.*

Your body has been operating on very little food, keeping you in motion by pulling from your fat stores. Once it begins receiving a more normal amount of food, it's likely to hang on for dear life to whatever you give it. In other words, you're more vulnerable to weight gain during Phase 3 than you would be ordinarily. Your body doesn't know that you are done with giving it so few calories to work with, so it's being smart and lowering your metabolism. Slowly returning fats and calories to your diet reduces the chance of regaining the weight.

If you go too quickly, your endocrine system will work hard to bring you back to your old, higher set point by increasing your hunger hormones and decreasing your metabolism. The body seeks homeostasis, so even if it would be healthiest for you to remain at the lower weight, your body thinks of your longstanding, higher weight as your "safe place." Going slowly reduces this effect.

2. *It protects your ketosis.*

Once you're no longer on the low calorie diet, testing your ketones will become important. This is true whether or not you want to begin a ketogenic diet, but it's extra valuable if you do.

You could measure ketones with urine strips, which indicate whether or not you're in ketosis (and roughly how deeply you are in it) or you could use a ketone/glucose meter, which tests the actual level of ketones in your blood. Meters give you a more precise reading, but the blood test strips they require are expensive.

As you re-introduce foods and increase calories during Phase 3, monitor your ketones, not just your weight. Slow your pace ...if you notice you are getting close to dipping out of ketosis; that would mean any less than a .5 reading on your monitor.

Important: Expect to have lower ketone levels as soon as you're done with the hormone; don't worry about that at all. HCG + fasting drives ketosis very strongly (and eating 500 calories is essentially a fast). We just want you to guard against dropping *out* of ketosis by taking it slow in P3.

3.   *It gives your digestive system time to re-adjust to fats.*

For the sake of your gall bladder, it's safest to ease back into consuming fats. That's true for everyone, but especially true for people who had a gall bladder that was compromised to begin with. Some people have had their gall bladder removed so are aware of their need for caution, but many people are unaware that they are vulnerable to a gall bladder attack. Perhaps they have a genetic marker for liver problems, have Type 2 diabetes, or have over-worked their digestive system by giving it too much fat over time. In any of these cases, your body would be overwhelmed by rapid re-introduction of fats. Going slow reduces the chance of a gall bladder attack.

4.   *It enables you to test for food sensitivities.*

While you were on Phase 2, you eliminated most of the foods you normally eat. If there are specific foods (or categories of food) you think your body reacts poorly to, Phase 3 is the time to test that theory. After all, you have already done an elimination diet!

For example, if you suspect your body doesn't tolerate fresh, young dairy very well (cottage cheese, sour cream, yogurt, ricotta, cream cheese, milk, whipping cream, kefir) eating these foods after not having had them for a long while will give you that answer. Does your stomach bloat? Do you get gassy? Develop dark circles under your eyes? Break out in acne? It's all so attractive. There's much more below about what symptoms to watch for when testing. Going slow is the only way to uncover food sensitivities, because you must test individual foods, one at a time.

During Phase 3, spend about a week in each "tier" of foods (below) slowly re-introducing things you enjoy but weren't able to eat during P2. You needn't eat anything you don't care for; the foods listed below are just examples of what you *could* re-introduce if you wanted to.

You may of course take it slower than one week per tier if you want to be extra careful about not regaining the weight you've lost, though most people are pretty eager to diversify their diet beyond turkey breast and celery once they reach Phase 3.

Even if you're not officially testing for food sensitivities, we suggest you be very observant during Phase 3. If you add just one new food each day, you'll know exactly what caused any symptoms you may have; keep notes so you don't lose this information! For example, if you were doing fine with egg whites during P2, then get a headache and become irritable when you begin eating whole eggs, you're likely reacting to egg yolks. (This experiment will not work if you are already a grouch.)

5.   *It decreases the possibility of weight rebound.*

After rapid or "intensive" weight loss (by any means, not just by HCG) people sometimes feel deprived and a little janky. Though they're delighted with what they've accomplished, they have missed the freedom to eat as much as they want. When people eat aggressively for a time, out of deprivation, it's called *weight rebound.*

To prevent weight rebound, you'll pace yourself extra conservatively during Phase 3. Familiarize yourself with the **Eating Guide to HCG Phase 3** that appears below so you can adhere to it. If you find you're experiencing rapid weight gain even while adhering to Phase 3, here are a few tweaks that should help:

— Be more gradual about increasing your calories. Add 100-200 calories every *other* day, rather than every day.

— Slow the rate at which you re-introduce new foods.

— Remain longer in each of the three tiers.

Within each tier Phase 3, add *one new food* per day to your diet, rather than allowing yourself everything in a particular category. For example, in Tier 1, the second category of foods is eggs and oily fish, like salmon. Ordinarily on P3, you could add both of these foods at the same time if you wanted to, but if weight rebound is a concern, choose just eggs or oily fish to re-introduce on a single day.

Eating Guide to HCG Phase 3

During HCG Phase 3, re-introduce foods one tier at a time.
Eat only foods you like. There are no particular foods required.

Increase 100-200 calories per day.
Stop increasing when you've reached your target number of calories for the maintenance stage. Generally this is a bit below your basal metabolic rate.

Spend roughly a week in each tier.
Spend longer if you are gaining weight. Spend longer if you're losing ketosis.

In Tiers 2 and 3, you needn't add foods in the precise order listed.
Decide the order based upon what you're eager to eat.

Tier 1 foods — HCG Phase 3

Healthy fats

Avocado, avocado oil, coconut oil, olive oil, grass-fed butter, cacao butter

Whole eggs, oily fish like salmon, black cod, sea bass or branzino

Organic fatty meats like pork belly, ribeye steak or short ribs
Fatty poultry like dark meat chicken or duck with skin

Tier 2 foods — HCG Phase 3

Higher-carb veggies than you ate on Phase 2 (but still no starchy vegetables)

Examples: Artichokes, olives, carrots, cherry tomatoes, spaghetti squash and larger portions of veggies that were on our suggested veggie tiers 3 and 4.

Aged (hard) dairy

Examples: Aged gouda, aged cheddar, cave aged gruyere, petit basque, parmesan, pecorino, romano, asiago cheeses.

Fresh (soft) dairy

Examples: Full-fat cottage cheese, full-fat ricotta, heavy whipping cream, mascarpone, brie, camembert, taleggio, other bloomy or washed-rind cheeses, bleu cheese, farmer's cheese, feta or cojito cheese, fresh mozzarella or burrata, paneer or haloumi cheese.

TIP: Try paneer or haloumi cheese sautéed in butter, ghee, olive oil, avocado oil, coconut oil or animal fat like chicken schmalz or pork lard. Paneer and haloumi become crisp rather than melting when pan fried!

Full fat yogurt

Try yogurt separately from other fresh dairy.

Tier 3 foods — HCG Phase 3

Lowest glycemic fruits

Examples: Raspberry, blackberry, strawberry, starfruit

Low glycemic fruits

Examples: Coconut, plum, kiwi, watermelon, cantaloupe, peach, clementine, blueberry

Lowest carb nuts and seeds

Examples: Pili nuts, pecans, macadamia nuts, brazil nuts, pumpkin seeds

Moderate carb nuts and seeds

Examples: hazelnuts, walnuts, almonds, pine nuts, sunflower seeds

Higher-carb fruit, vegetables, nuts and seeds
(only for people who are not transitioning to keto)

Fruit examples: Apple, pineapple, mango, pomegranate, nectarine
Veggie examples: Butternut squash, beets, parsnips, shallots, yams
Nut and seed examples: Pistachios, cashews, quinoa

Continuing a Ketogenic Lifestyle

The HCG Diet is a special project: it's a diet, not a lifestyle. HCG is not intended to be sustainable. If you choose to maintain ketogenic eating after HCG, *that's* a lifestyle.

Eating "keto" is not about food lists and calorie counting; it's about low carbohydrate eating for a lifetime. What the HCG Diet has in common with a ketogenic lifestyle is that both benefit from your creativity and your attention to detail. The other, more literal connection between them is that being on HCG puts you in ketosis and eating keto keeps you there.

Both the HCG Diet and a ketogenic lifestyle are about accelerated fat burning. When you were on HCG, you were in nutritional ketosis. During this time, the hormone helped you burn stored fat much more efficiently than you would normally. You may choose to continue being in ketosis, if you would like. You would accomplish this by eating a diet very low in carbohydrate, moderate in protein and sufficient in healthy, non-inflammatory fats to keep you satiated. The ketogenic diet (1) minimizes the sugars and starches you consume. This sharp reduction in carbohydrate then (2) shifts your body from burning glucose for fuel to burning fat. Both of these tasks have already been accomplished by people just completing the HCG Diet. HCG provides a very natural running start to the ketogenic diet.

What's special about HCG as a springboard to keto, though, is that the human chorionic gonadotropin hormone puts you in an unusually deep state of ketosis. Whereas some people struggle to get into mild ketosis when they begin keto, particularly if they are beginning the project with high blood sugar, people coming to keto from HCG are in deep ketosis; their body has already made the shift to fat burning mode.

Those starting keto from scratch also have the work of sharply decreasing their carbohydrate intake for a stretch, which people on the HCG Diet have already accomplished. Some patients also need to add a period of building healthy fats into their diet (which people on HCG already did in Phase 3) or they take exogenous ketone supplements in an effort to achieve ketosis. People who've begun keto by doing HCG don't need to worry about either of these things.

What if you were to take human chorionic gonadotropin without actually doing a low calorie HCG diet? If you ate too many carbs, you would *not* go into ketosis. HCG does not magically drop you into ketosis. We think it mobilizes fat stores — though research is ongoing — but we know for sure that it tickles the hypothalamus, reducing hunger signals. This combination of effects is very useful for losing fat on the HCG Diet, but sharply reduced carbohydrate intake *must* occur for ketosis to kick in.

What if you did the Loading Phase of the HCG Diet but not the low calorie phase? Yes, if you practiced loading in the way we describe here (low carb, moderate protein, high fat) the HCG hormone would help put you into ketosis, but actually continuing on to the low calorie phase drives ketosis further. We cannot know what would be healthiest for you personally, but here are some considerations that should weigh on your decision:

1. Dr. Simeons in his original protocol warns against patients being on HCG for less than 23 days. This argues against using the Loading Phase just to get into ketosis.

2. Some patients are not advised to lose weight. This argues against requiring 23 days on a low calorie diet. For these people, a loading phase and then a nutritionally sound ketogenic diet (without the HCG diet) might be fine.

HCG for Foodies is geared to the reader who (1) will in fact complete the HCG Diet protocol, with professional supervision and (2) for whom it is medically and psychologically safe to do so. With these conditions met, using HCG to transition to keto is likely an excellent choice.

If you plan to continue eating for ketosis after HCG Phase 3, you will not return grains, starchy vegetables, beans, legumes, high glycemic fruits or sugars to your diet, at least not in the typical amounts. This may sound restrictive, but many patients find that there are so many delicious low carbohydrate dishes to prepare that "eating keto" actually amounts to an increase in their quality of life.

Eating keto calls for a major shift in attitude towards what's healthy; many who have adopted it refer to choosing a *ketogenic lifestyle*. This is an apt description, in our opinion, since developing a talent for advance planning is a huge element of success on keto. For example, learning to make low carb versions of high carb favorites like waffles and tortillas requires planning and effort, as does collecting tasty low-carb snacks for work and travel, prepping enough of a dish to last several meals and bringing keto desserts to potluck gatherings. All of these behaviors are common practice for people who have adopted a ketogenic lifestyle.

As with the HCG Diet, when you would on occasion have just egg whites for breakfast or just tuna for lunch, people on keto may find that they benefit from adjusting what they think of as a normal meal. Rather than the protein + starch side dish + cooked vegetable meals many of us grew up with, experienced people on keto might have a big bowl of egg salad with homemade mayonnaise for breakfast, roasted Brussels sprouts with bacon for lunch and a ribeye steak with butter or bleu cheese for dinner. As we've discussed, adjusting your perspective is all it takes to spark behavior change. For more on understanding the psychology of successful transition, jump ahead to "How Behavior Change Works."

Consider leveraging your fat burning during HCG for a quick start to the long-term fat burning of ketosis. If you decide to continue on to eating ketogenic, *pay special attention during Phase 3 to returning fats and proteins to your diet but leaving out high carbohydrate foods*, even if they are considered safe in general for P3. For example, many people re-introduce sweet potatoes or yams at the end of HCG Phase 3, but you would not do this if you wanted to remain in ketosis.

If you go keto, you'll likely find a supportive community of people who have learned ingenious workarounds for high carb foods and who are seeing clinical improvement of diabetes and other metabolic disorders. These patients report feeling healthier and more energetic in a variety of ways — including but not limited to weight loss.

As with any change that will be visible to others, being good-humored but assertive about your choices is vital to your success. If someone offers you a baked potato with bacon bits and sour cream, and you are eating low carbohydrate, you'll have to be brave enough to joke that you eat bacon bits and sour cream, but not potato. If you deliver assertiveness with a sense of humor, others will understand that you're serious.

If you decide to adopt a ketogenic lifestyle, don't skip past the section on "Interpersonal Skills for Transitions" in this book. Most people are absolutely delighted by the vast benefits of eating low carbohydrate, but also say that dealing with other people can be a challenge. Patients say that responding to everything from sincere questions to rude challenges shakes them up. We hope you'll go for the lifelong benefits of a ketogenic eating and will prepare for those conversations.

What we've described is the rationale for using the HCG Diet to jumpstart the Ketogenic Diet. If you'd like all the information you'd need to actually embark on a ketogenic lifestyle, we recommend you read *Keto.* by Maria Emmerich & Craig Emmerich.

Guide to Testing Food Sensitivities

Using Phase 3 to test for food sensitivities is entirely optional; it's a matter of choice that some people have little patience for after suffering through P2. Observing your food sensitivities would require you to be careful about introducing *one new food every two days*, so if you do have symptoms, you'll know precisely which food is to blame.

After many weeks of skinless chicken breast, it's probably hard to imagine adding just one new food at a time, 100-200 calories at a time. Many patients do speed through Phase 3 because they are eager to eat freely again. For example, they bring dairy and whole eggs back at the same time, losing valuable information about how their body responds to each of those ingredients individually.

Do your best to treat Phase 3 as an "elimination and challenge diet." This means that you observe closely how your body handles the challenge of each new food you re-introduce to your diet.

If there's a particular food (or category of foods) you have a strong hunch about, investigating it now would be worth your while. You have already done the hard part: eliminating that food entirely from your diet for a month or so. Now, when you eat several portions of that food in a row, if your body has a reaction it will really let you know.

Why is testing food sensitivities relevant to maintaining your weight loss? Because foods that our body doesn't tolerate well cause inflammation. Systemic inflammation slows or stalls weight loss.

If you decide to investigate your possible food sensitivities during HCG Phase 3, here's how to do it:

Day 1: Introduce a new food, eating it at least 3 times throughout the day. Be alert to any signs of an immediate food sensitivity; the list of symptoms is below. If you discover a bodily reaction, make a note of your observations and stop eating that food. If there's no reaction, you will continue watching for reactions on Day 2.

Note: In the first several weeks of HCG Phase 3, you're still not eating many calories. It may be difficult to eat large portions of the food you're testing, so prioritize having small amounts of that food at three points on Day 1 of testing.

Day 2: If no reaction to a food on Day 1, *don't* eat it again on Day 2, just continue looking for possible reactions to the food, including a marked weight increase this morning. Write your observations.

Day 3: When you wake up and weigh yourself on Day 3, if you've still observed no symptoms in response to this food, including no sudden weight gain, it's very unlikely that food will cause you inflammation. It's safe to incorporate this food in your post-HCG diet.

Any foods you do note a sensitivity to, set aside until you've completed Phase 3, at minimum. Since your body doesn't tolerate that food gracefully, it's a threat to stabilizing your weight.

Symptoms of a Food Sensitivity

Abrupt gain of roughly two or more pounds
Hard, bloated belly
Heartburn or acid reflux
Flatulence or loose stool

Feeling slightly nauseous, feeling "a little off"
Fatigue or sleepiness after eating

Face or ears flush, feel warm
Rash
Acne

Post nasal drip
Stuffy nose
Headache
Watery or goopy eyes
Dark circles under eyes

Difficulty stopping once you start eating that food
Increased appetite or cravings
Sudden urge to discuss politics

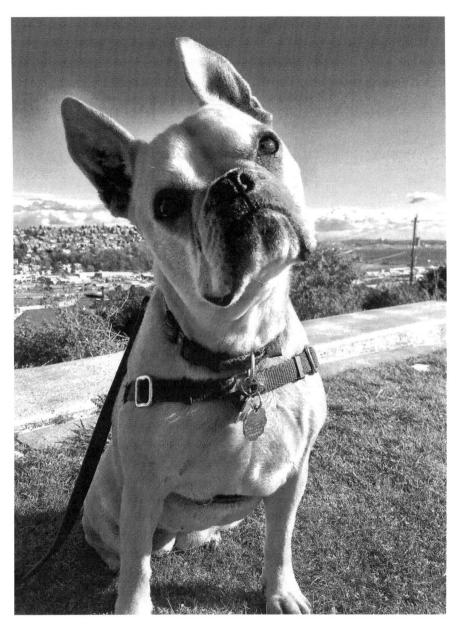

Photo: Dana Falk

Babette develops goop in her eyes and dark circles beneath them whenever she eats poultry. We all have some foods our body doesn't tolerate well, but we have to look for clues.

The symptoms above are not an exhaustive list! Just be alert to physical changes when you eat a lot of something you haven't had in a long time.

With some of the foods you test, it won't seem 100% clear whether you had a reaction or not; perhaps you experienced mild heartburn or a slight rash. Any foods you *suspect* a sensitivity to, just set aside until you've completed P3. You'll want to prevent any threat to stabilizing your new weight. If you didn't have a rash at all, then you ate a lot of olives one day, and now you have a mild rash — just assume that's a reaction to olives.

For much more detailed information about individual reactions to food, read *Food Allergies and Food Intolerance: The Complete Guide to their Identification and Treatment* by Brostoff and Gamlin (2000). It's easy to find an inexpensive, used copy of this excellent book.

How Behavior Change Works

Some people get invested in projects only after they have examined the underlying theory. These people buy-in and take action only after they understand how things work. Other people prefer to dive in, take action and not worry about why or how; they don't particularly need to understand the underlying process. The next few sections are for readers who want to understand the psychology of behavior change, because they know these insights will improve their success with the diet.

Ambivalence is powerful

We don't always realize when we have changed our minds about wanting to do something. Sigmund Freud wrote in The Psychopathology of Everyday Life (1901) *"...Intentions of some importance are 'forgotten' when obscure motives arise to disturb them...."* In other words, we unconsciously abandon our goals were when we're not entirely on board. We're still telling ourselves that we intend to take action, but deep down, our priorities have shifted and we're no longer motivated enough to actually do it.

Some people have great insight about their own personality: they realize that they keep "prioritizing other goals" so that the toughest or most unpleasant things never quite happen. Usually our ambivalence is hidden from us, though, and it's a more powerful force because of that. Here's a basic principle of human psychology: when something we were unconscious of becomes conscious, we have much more control over it. Self-awareness is incredibly useful.

Ambivalence means that we get attached to the idea of something being a valuable challenge, and to thinking of ourselves as the kind of person who loves a good challenge, but we are not actually eager enough to follow-through. We want the outcome but don't realize that we're not up for the work.

This whole thing should sound pretty familiar — we've all done it. We haven't admitted to ourselves "...I don't really *want* the work of quitting smoking / going back to work or school / changing careers / losing weight / living on a budget / raising children / caring for a pet..." but we are still carrying on with the assumption that we do want to make the change. We believe we are somewhere in the process of change; it's a story we like and we're hanging on to it.

So here's one positive aspect of the challenges the HCG diet presents: you will have to decide whether you want to push past whatever reservations you've had about losing weight. If you do this diet well, or even relatively well, you will lose serious weight. As we've discussed, P2 requires planning and shopping, social assertiveness, creativity, time, money and sheer strength. It will almost certainly mean some periods of hunger, boredom and fatigue. You will eat egg whites when you really want a cheese omelette and eat baked fish when you really want fish and chips. You've got to want the work, not just the outcome.

If you blow off facing ambivalence while taking the HCG hormone, you may *gain* weight. This is no time for half-assing it, because eating normally when your body is so hyper-sensitive to fat and carbohydrate can cause a jump in weight. Taking action may feel sort of liberating: you're done with the tiresome decision-making stage and on to taking action. In therapy, it's common for people to say that finally making a decision they've been dancing around feels really good, even if that means they've decided to *abandon* a goal. That's how much power ambivalence has!

The Psychology research on ambivalence towards behavior change is really interesting. Most people who want to make some lifestyle change have aspects of the new behavior they are worried about. What other people would think of them is a common concern. Other times the concern is that making a change would mean they are not being themselves, not being authentic. This vague worry may create just enough resistance that the change never takes flight.

Ambivalence is remarkable. If you ask a person trying to quit smoking, "...Are you still deciding about quitting...?" they will usually say, "...Not at all! I really want to quit and have for some time...." But if you were to give them a questionnaire asking the pros and cons of making this change, their score often shows that they see just enough cons to let the project fall away. They have *just enough hesitation* to not fully meet the challenge.

This part is important: Research shows that we can't just "feel more positive than negative" about making a change for us to kick into gear. We have to feel *significantly* more positive about the work and emotional risk of change than we feel anxious or negative about it (Prochaska, Norcross & DiClemente, 1994.)

In their terrific book *Changing for Good,* Prochaska, Norcross and DiClemente studied subjects who said they wanted to make a major life change. When they asked subjects in multiple studies about their concerns with making this life change, they discovered that people are often more ambivalent about their goals than they had realized. Only subjects who could think of *far more benefits than costs* to making a behavior change took all the emotional, planning and action steps necessary for lasting change.

Don't we all fear calling attention to ourselves or inconveniencing others? Seeming needy or seeming selfish? Exerting too much energy or wasting too much time? Don't we simply fear failing? When we make a list of pros and cons, we may assume that whichever list is longest wins. It turns out that's often not true. It may be that you *do* want to lose weight, but there are one or two hesitations that are powerful disincentives. What might those be?

It's quite common for people to use therapy to dig for these insights. Any time you're not actually making plans for something you thought you always wanted, suspect ambivalence. Sometimes it's simply that a time crunch has meant we prioritize short-term needs and lose long-term goals, but often it's more complex than that.

If you'd like a deeper dive into the ambivalence some people feel about a slimmer body, jump ahead to the section called "Why People Fear Weight Loss."

Formula for Lasting Change

We each have a personality. Each of us tends to prefer either (1) reflecting on our needs, (2) thinking plans through in detail or (3) taking physical action. The problem is, we need patience for all three of these skills to create lasting change.

— Some people think about things for too long and don't fully take action. They have reflected on their life to this point and allowed themselves to feel what they've missed out on. They understand themselves well and have decided they want the change, but they don't ever formulate a plan of action. That part seems unnecessary to them. "...If I want it enough, I'll make it happen..." *Thinking without action usually results in smaller-scale changes than hoped-for.*

— Some people leap to action without having contemplated their feelings or made a plan. They are impatient with the reflection and the preparation. They may think all that's a waste of time and feel eager to dive into a behavior change. *Action without planning usually leads to temporary change that backslides.* Making a change and then realizing you can't maintain those results is maddening, but still people try to take action without having strategized! This makes people wonder if even trying to change is futile.

— The key to making a major lifestyle change that will stick is Contemplation + Preparation + Action = lasting change. There's exceptionally strong research to support these observations, by Prochaska, Norcross & DiClemente (1994). If you want to lose weight and keep it off, you'll want to spend time with the emotional experiences that compel you to do this (Contemplation) + work in advance on how you will have what you need and how you'll avoid unnecessary challenges to your goals (Preparation) + systematically carry out your plan of action, making whatever sacrifices of time, money, energy, bravery are required (Action).

This is a vast over-simplification of a great book, *Changing for Good.* Check it out if you want to be very intentional about your desire to get healthy. Their principles work for engineering any kind of behavior change. (In fact, weight loss is not even a focus of the book.) Buy it used and highlight the hell out if it.

Create allies

Once people do take action, we know that *telling others about the change they're working on increases their chances of success.* Inventing excuses to cover for some new behavior you've developed is a drag, but the real reason 'being out' is an advantage is that it gives other people an opportunity to be your ally. For example, if the behavior someone was changing was to eat vegetarian, and he or she has been invited to a barbecue, they're more likely to succeed if they've told the hosts. That way, the hosts can think about whether they'd like to put something on the grill that a vegetarian would enjoy. Perhaps when they shop for groceries they will grab a few portobello mushrooms or some field roast hot dogs to put on the grill for anyone who might prefer them. They might also decide to leave the bacon out of the pasta salad or to set some pasta aside before they put the bacon in. Not everyone is accommodating — heck, some people are downright odd when others make a dietary change — but giving friends an opportunity to be an ally is a wise choice.

As for you on HCG, when friends are given a heads-up about what you're doing, it reduces the chances they will feel offended that you didn't eat what they made. It also gives them an opportunity to rise to the occasion and that's nice to think about. Research shows clearly that part of your preparation for a diet should be to let some people know what you're up to.

Even if you are 'out' about being on HCG, you may want to bring an extra **portobello mushroom cap marinated in lime zest and jalapeño** to share with other guests at the barbecue. Having something tasty to put on the grill (and enough of it to share) prevents your diet from disrupting the party.

It's the interpersonal aspect of HCG that worries people. Let's be frank: there *are* people whose personality may make this a challenge. There are loudmouths who will declare anything they don't understand to be bullshit. There are sweet, inquisitive people who will ask for more detail than they should. There are compulsive debaters who will try to pick apart the logic of any idea that wasn't theirs. There are amateur nutritionists who will try to teach how you should *really* lose weight. There's an entire section later in this book on "Interpersonal Skills for Transitions" that may be useful to you.

Change inspires change

People have a tendency to change more than one thing in their lives at a time. Somehow we feel mobilized, energized. Seemingly unrelated areas of our lives may get unstuck, which is neat to think about. For example, some patients say that as they began to eat more thoughtfully, they also began to research a possible career change / complete the paperwork for an adoption or a passport / repair things that are broken / get their finances in order and such. Enjoy the fruits of your labor. This is likely to be a bigger, more liberating change than you'd imagined.

You can work the other end of the equation, too. What changes have you already made that might liberate you to lose weight? Did you finally ask for a promotion? Leave an unhappy relationship? Clean your living space? Manage alcohol or other substances? Admit to an error? Finally get help with your taxes? Finally travel alone? If so, why not leverage that success to work on losing weight?

It's so interesting, given how consistent our personalities are across a lifetime, that we can change an attitude we've long held. In response to just one life transition, we can decide we think or feel differently about a position. We can actually change what we *want* and what we *believe*, in response to something we *do*.

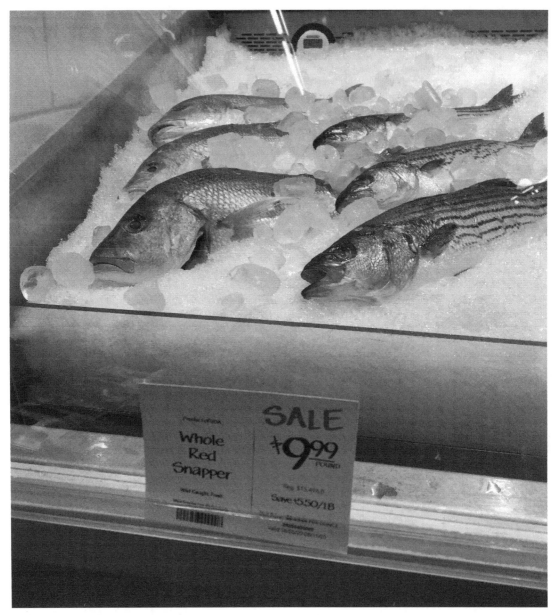

Photo: Dana Falk

You never used to notice the whole fish on ice, but now you know several ways to prepare fresh red snapper! Now, you think that people who skip the whole fish are missing out. Behavior can lead and attitudes follow.

Once people see that they get what they wanted, due to planning and effort, they're on a roll. For example, once people begin to get organized, they often have disdain for people who don't have their act together. Their attitude is now that being well-organized is a virtue.

Once someone makes a change, they are now in a club of sorts! That club might be people who pay their bills on time. People who exercise regularly. People who are getting a degree. People who attend spiritual services. People who take care of themselves. People who grocery shop thoughtfully. *It's true that attitudes change and behaviors follow, but it also works the other way around. Behavior can lead and belief will follow.* Change creates more change.

It's skill, not luck

Changing patterns doesn't have much to do with luck. *Sometimes we get lucky about favorable circumstances, but lifelong behavior change is deliberate and strategic.* It's you who must mastermind those strategies and who must personalize them to play to your strengths. That requires both planning skills (this section) and self-awareness skills (the next section).

If you are a person who tends to deal with anxiety by telling yourself "...*Whatever is meant to happen to me will happen naturally...*" you are focused on good fortune. It's true that there's an element of luck to our metabolic health. Some people have diabetes in the family, or a naturally larger frame or a family in which nutrition was not within reach and some other people had none of these disadvantages. Luck is not the most productive focus, though.

When following a rigorous diet like HCG, your success will hinge mostly on your skills. You'll use time management skills to make sure you shop for ingredients and interpersonal skills to defend your picky eating. You'll use motivation skills to track every bite you eat for several weeks and intellectual skills to remember the science of how weight loss fluctuates. You'll use patience to research the various foods you might eat on HCG and planning skills to have prepared meals in the freezer. If you put in the work, you'll have a lot to be proud of.

The way you'll eat on the HCG Diet is not meant to be sustainable. We'll focus next on a few tactics for a making a rather extreme, short-term behavior change such as what the HCG Diet calls for.

If you'd like to geek-out on diverse strategies for lasting behavior change, read Gretchen Rubin's (2018) excellent book *Better Than Before: Mastering the habits of our everyday lives*. She embarked on major research to pull together an inspiring variety of tactics you might employ to make a change stick.

Tactics for Changing a Short-Term Behavior

Clear your calendar

Don't make social plans during the time you're on Phase 2 if you can help it. Try to spend time with friends focused on common activities or good conversation rather than meal time. Put off events that may feel like a challenge to your eating for the 3-5 weeks you're on HCG. It may seem intense to clear your calendar around a diet, but it's for a short period, during which the challenge and the payoff are both high. It's the same thing people do when they're in Finals Week or they're about to move across country or they have a newborn baby or an older person who needs their care: they set other things aside for a little while. Most people find that laying low while they are eating so few calories is helpful, so they guard their calendar during this time.

Study the diet protocol like crazy

Whether you're following the original Simeons protocol to the letter or adapting it in the ways we suggest, you have got to know the HCG Diet backwards and forwards. How many days do you eat high fat before switching to low fat? What vegetables are on the original protocol? How should you handle breakfast? Is there a rule about lemons? Eggs? How many grams of protein are recommended? Can you drink a can of diet soda? You should know this stuff inside-out.

If you are serious about being tactical, you'll need to build your familiarity with the material at hand. This would be equally true if your goal were to get better at managing your personal finances, for example. You might read about credit card debt, take an online class in budgeting or study the book *Personal Finance for Dummies*. You might listen to podcasts about personal finance hosted by credentialed professionals or might consult in person with a Certified Financial Planner. You might go to the library for a book on how to improve your credit score or attend a workshop on this topic. Without a knowledge base, we are casting about, hoping for a good outcome with only a vague sense of how it works.

Early in this book there's a section called "Old Protocol and New Advances" that is too long to tattoo on the back of your hand, but it's that important. Equally important are the sections "Method for Choosing Fruits and Vegetables" and "Method for Choosing Proteins." We recommend you study this diet protocol like crazy.

Keep track of relevant data

You probably know that monitoring the details of any behavior makes it more likely you'll accomplish your goals. *Even if the research didn't demonstrate it so convincingly, you'd probably know that we do better when we monitor progress.* Monitoring is a two-part strategy: (1) you must decide which details to focus on, then (2) you must take the time to keep track of those numbers.

The data you track is up to you, but here are some ideas:

— Calories consumed
— Grams of carbohydrate consumed
— Ounces of water drunk
— Amount of MCT oil and tummy response
— Foods that made you retain water
— Scale weight
— Waist circumference

— Measurement of hips, neck, upper arms, upper thighs, etc.
— How well you're sleeping
— Time you started /stopped eating each day ("eating window")

Some people track just the bare bones — calories consumed and scale weight — others will add interesting data, such as keeping a list of the foods they find satisfying, keeping a log of how their mood changes as they lose weight or measuring how many reps of walking around the block they can do in a day. We do recommend that you at least take a few body measurements *at the very beginning of the process.* This will help you to appreciate that on some days, the scale doesn't move but your body is losing fat.

In order to track relevant data, you'll have to either make a computer spreadsheet, use a phone application or bust out some old-school graph paper. Your relationship to technology doesn't matter; you have got to generate data. Jump back to the section "Video, Recipe and Workbook Resources" for details on a workbook by HCG Chica that helps you track your data.

Challenge yourself to gather data even if fussing with details or numbers is not your usual style. You will be so glad that you can look back and see how you spent your calories and whether you like what you see. For example, some people choose to have egg whites for breakfast. It's not super delicious, but an egg white is only 17 calories! The protein in two egg whites would stop your belly growling for several hours. That's a pretty great investment of 34 calories. **Add some spinach and mushrooms to the egg whites** and now you've got something quite palatable for about 50 calories.

On the other hand, you might look back at the egg white breakfast a few days later and realize that you have had trouble controlling eating at lunch because you hated your low calorie breakfast. In that case, maybe you will decide to spread your calories more evenly throughout the day, so you won't feel deprived.

Tracking data is important because it's illuminating; it enables you to shift your approach midstream.

Pack what you need, wherever you go

Your best bet while on HCG is to bring along whatever supplies you'll need to meet your immediate goals. Don't be afraid to look like a dweeb: bring your own snacks for long drives, meetings, parties, travel, movies, ballgames, conferences and anything else that would take you away from home. Don't assume that any given catered meal, restaurant or convenience store will have what you need. Bring **cans of Zevia iced tea, zipper bags of jerky, a crunchy bell pepper.** Bring **tiny containers of MCT oil,** perhaps even a scale for weighing your proteins. You will be the person with a **hard boiled egg** in your bag and a little **packet of PGX fiber** in your pocket. So what? Once you are on Phase 3, when you are increasing calories, fats and types of food, eating away from home will become much easier, but for Phase 2, pack what you need.

Reward yourself in a different area of life

Noticing smaller successes *en route* to a larger goal is a productive approach to change in adulthood. We reward smaller, intermediate accomplishments along the way to a larger goal — called "successive approximations" in Psychology — when we potty train kids, house train dogs, recognize employee performance and all the rest. The trick now, on HCG, is for you to notice your own mini-successes and choose something you'd like as a reward other than food.

Both parts of this homework are difficult: (1) noticing our mini-successes and (2) choosing something other than food to celebrate them with. Food is a natural treat for us, just as it is for dogs. With advanced dog training, as with advanced tactics for human behavior change, we discontinue the use of edible treats and reward the dog with a walk, a toy, a scratch, even with tone of voice.

Examples of rewarding yourself with something other than food:

— Buy a new release movie rather than just watching what comes with your streaming subscription.

— Work on a home improvement project

— Go to a park you've never explored

— Create a music playlist

— Think of a phrase you'd like to be able to say in ten languages, then learn to do that

— Call a long-distance friend or relative

— Play with a pet

— Take a mid-day nap

— Go for a drive

— Order something for your home that's completely your taste

— Buy an article of clothing or a grooming product that's new to you

— Take a bath or shower

— Buy something practical you've been needing

— Plant something that's symbolic of your growth

— Plan or fantasize about some travel

— Read or write a book

— Organize a cupboard or drawer

— Play an instrument or learn to play one

— Work on a craft

— Go to a thrift store and see what oddity you can find for just a few dollars

— Write a thank you note to someone who is supporting you

Reward yourself with anything from a tiny pot of chives on the windowsill to a beautiful Japanese maple planted in the yard. The point is that you learn to reward yourself for intermediate goals, not just grand ones, and that you discover treats other than food.

Bonus points if you choose a reward that's related to your weight loss goals. For example, make a music playlist you'd like to exercise to. Buy large bins for organizing clothes that are too big and too small for you. Call a friend or relative who is likely to motivate you or who listens well. Set up a cozy corner of your home for reading, writing, tracking your diet.

Match your strategies to your styles

It's easy to find advice for behavior change, but it's up to you to know what would work for you personally. You will adapt strategies to your style, like we all do. *The briefer your round of HCG, the more vital it is that you already know what tactics work best for you.* The next section, "Personal Insights Useful for Weight Loss," will walk you through this process.

Perhaps other people succeed with variety in their day, but you personally do better with repetition. Other people may appreciate time with friends when they're concentrating on a project, but you may prefer time alone when working on something difficult. Other people may like to reflect upon and write about body image issues, but you may prefer to reflect less and distract yourself with other interests. Other people may find that acquaintances rooting for them improves their success, but you may prefer rigorous questioning of your plan. Other people may prefer to have things mapped out, but you may prefer to figure things out as you go.

What is your personality style when you are working on a difficult project? Variety or repetition? Company or privacy? Reflection or distraction? Support or challenge? Planning or improvising? These insights may be applied to your strategy for the HCG Diet.

Interpersonal Skills for Transitions

Making behavior changes that stick isn't just about what you do, it's about how others respond to what you do. We suggest you rehearse for the intellectual and emotional challenges of making your needs known during this time. Dealing skillfully with others is vital to your success. Ask anyone who has to tell people that they do not drink alcohol, the their child has a nut allergy or who needs an accommodation at school or work... when you need something, your approach matters.

Appreciate the awkwardness for others

There's a funky dynamic when someone who has been overweight tries to lose weight. Some people in their lives may feel awkward about encouraging their efforts, because it may make them feel trapped into acknowledging that person has weight to lose.

It's a double-bind for them, so you may get some skittish responses. Show them how to respond by describing your philosophy: don't call this a 'crash diet' or be critical of your body. You can simply say that you've decided to undertake something very positive for your health — your metabolic health, your cardiac health, your complexion, your digestion, your physical energy — and losing weight would help with all of these things. Anyone can comfortably endorse you wanting to be healthier overall, right? You're not saying that you are flawed or that *they* should do what you are doing; you're just saying that you deserve to be as healthy as possible and have decided to go for it.

This may get the other person thinking about a positive change for their own life, but that's not the point. The point is that you don't want them to feel that supporting your diet will offend you. Help these poor people with the double-bind: frame your HCG project as something that is more important (and more interesting) than simply wanting to wear a smaller size.

HCG is legit; you deserve respect

Some people observe lent, ramadan or passover by making behavior changes. You would show respect for their practice even if it's not what you do, right? The same is true for your round of HCG: you deserve respect for the changes you're making, even from people who don't understand the process — but you may need to explain that what you're doing is not bullshit.

Friends and family are right to be concerned if they hear that someone they love is eating very few calories. If someone did not understand the science or that this is short-term, HCG *would* sound like a crash diet or an eating disorder. Thank them for being alert to your health.

You don't have to teach people the science underlying HCG unless you want to, but explanations of ketosis appear all over this book partly for that reason. If you want to give information without really discussing it, point them to the section "Note to Healthcare Professionals." The reasons HCG helps people burn fat is explained more colorfully in other sections of the book, but if you want info all in one place, with research citations, that is where to find it.

If you do want to teach people close to you about what you've embarked upon, you might explain that a natural hormone induces natural fat burning, but that the trade-off is your body is over-sensitive to any fat or carbohydrate you eat right now. That's why you're being so careful. You would point out that this is an established protocol with medical supervision. You'd share that it's a plan that typically yields great results, but then it will be up to you to continue eating well after you're done with the diet. Saying out loud that you don't expect all the work of getting healthy to be done with a short, intense diet may help relax their worries or judgment. This is actually a long-term project that begins with a special, short-term diet.

It's also true that some people don't mean to be insulting or dismissive, they are just sick of hearing about people's special dietary needs. One friend is gluten-free, even though they don't have celiac disease. Another friend is vegan for political reasons. One kid can have tree nuts but not peanuts. Your niece will only eat meat that's grass-fed. One co-worker is on a low fat / low sodium diet, another is on high fat / low carbohydrate diet. Your aunt will eat anything, but tracks points, calories or macronutrients. Understandably, some people are done having compassion for every special dietary need. In essence, they are questioning diets in general, not yours in particular.

Who is the freak?

Let's say you decline a friend's invitation to eat lunch out, because you're in HCG Phase 2, but you invite that friend to come to your place instead, so you can cook something for both of you. That would be a rather elegant and generous solution. What would you think of that friend if (s)he gave you a hard time about it? You might trust him or her less, going forward. You might feel manipulated or distanced. You might simply enjoy them less than you did before you saw this side of their personality.

If you wish, you may continue to propose solutions to the lunch impasse — for example, eating lunch out at a place that has a salad bar — but really, hasn't their response already changed your regard for the friend a bit? Are *you* the freak, for needing to eat carefully for a few months, or is it the person who cannot be flexible enough to come to your house for lunch?

You do not need to valiantly seek middle ground about where to eat when you're on HCG. Ultimately, if a friend keeps pushing back, it may be wise to hold off on making lunch plans at all with that person until you're at least to Phase 3 of the diet. People wearing a leg cast don't usually make plans for a hike until they're walking more comfortably.

Bottom line: *any time you are invited to do something that would set you back on your goals, and you propose an alternative, that's a show of self-respect.* If the other person is accommodating, that's a show of respect for you. If they're not, re-scheduling plans might be wisest.

Do your thing even if it annoys people

As you work through losing weight, you will probably notice:
— who is supporting you enthusiastically
— who has a few questions but is rooting for you
— who is skeptical about the diet but open to learning more
— who is critical of you or the diet without a desire to learn more

Someone who is critical of your HCG project but not curious about it may be sending the message, "*...That sounds dumb. Why bother...?*" That message may be completely unintended, but frankly, sometimes it is intended.

If that person is self-centered enough, (s)he may even try to convince you that you're not important enough to have goals, or that they are a better judge of what is worthwhile than you are. In other words, your new focus on health is inconvenient for them, frustrating for them or threatening to them. Interestingly, even criticism from people we don't respect can affect our mood and confidence! It's weird, but it's true.

Being on HCG is something special for you. Defend it tenaciously. Here are a variety of approaches to consider should you need to defend what you're doing:

— You can defend your project **proactively**, by suggesting places to meet that will work for you, like a farmer's market instead of a restaurant, or a walk instead of a meal.

— You can defend your project **graciously**, by kindly explaining your decision to do a tough diet and your optimism about the outcome.

— You can defend your project **quietly**, by saying nothing much when people question you, but resolutely continuing your dietary choices.

— You can defend your project **confrontationally**, by engaging in debate about hormonal weight loss and educating people about ketosis.

— You can defend your project **strategically**, by lying about why you are eating carefully. You could say you're investigating your food allergies and are doing an elimination diet.

However you approach a challenging conversation, your *behavior* can remain the same. You will be weighing your chicken breast for the next few weeks, even if someone else thinks that's dumb. When you have huge bags of clothes to donate to charity because they're too big to wear, you'll be entitled to feel smug.

Do your thing even if annoys other people. Remember, some people debate any idea they don't understand; it's just how their personality is constructed.

Some people debate compulsively

You know some people who argue as a reflex, don't you? Any concept they're unfamiliar with they call ridiculous. Any plan that wasn't their idea is stupid. Any project undertaken without their input is a waste of time. One might call that egotistical or aggressive, but in Psychology it's called "defensive minimization." This means trying to minimize the value given to something in order to protect one's status. (Sometimes this is their imagined status!)

For example, some people need to feel dominant and expert. To protect this status, they debate without much conscious thought. They diminish ideas and people that threaten their control, hoping that making someone else feel small will make them feel big. There are some mental health diagnoses associated with the use of defensive minimization and constant debate, but we won't venture there. Just know that you don't have to engage in any conversation that carries a sharp or dismissive tone. Trying to have a sincere conversation with someone who does nothing but debate is fruitless. Learning something is much more challenging for them than conflict is.

People who debate compulsively are sometimes able to be supportive if given a *very specific task* you'd like their assistance with. What drives them is the desire to be competent, authoritative, useful; to "know best" what will work. If you want them in your corner, tell them what specifically they could *do* that would make them indispensable.

You might say, "...*What I'm doing is difficult and your help would mean a lot to me. You are so good at making things work. When I need some special groceries, would you get them for me? Something that's a little hard to find, like purple cauliflower or MCT oil...?*"

Or you might say, "...*Instead of challenging why I'm doing this, could you ask me questions about how I will do it? I could use your help analyzing my project and planning for rough spots. You're such a good problem-solver....*"

Not everyone who uses conflict to establish their dominance can be soothed by giving them a job to do, but it's worth a try in some cases. Most often, the root of the problem for compulsive debaters is that they believe their competence is being challenged. They're unable to simply say, "…That's interesting. I've never heard of it. How does it work?…" Without the ability to tolerate not knowing something, and without the ability to soothe themselves, they lash out when asked to make a change for someone else, however small that change would be. It feels as though the person asking for a favor is trying to dominate them. Perhaps you already know someone whose personality is like that?

If someone you'll be dealing with while on HCG has a combative personality, your best bet may be to listen calmly to their debate but not correct them. Let them express themselves fully and without interruption. *Once they feel they've had their say, people usually de-escalate.* Then you can gradually change the subject, while you continue to *do what you need to do* for your round of HCG.

Relationship roles may shift

If you live with someone, and that person is accustomed to you preparing most of the meals, you may have some strategizing to do. Preparing meals that you cannot eat would not be fun. Switching up that expectation (at least while you're on HCG) would mean a shift of roles.

Here are some options to consider discussing with the person(s) accustomed to you doing most of the cooking. You might:

(1) Feed everyone in your home HCG-friendly meals while you're on P2;

(2) Prepare HCG meals for yourself. Someone else in the house old enough to cook can make their own non-HCG food;

(3) Make HCG meals for yourself as well as non-HCG meals for others, but mark the ingredients/dishes you have prepped for yourself so others will know they should save these only for you.

However you choose to handle cooking in the home, just make sure that your own meals are HCG-friendly.

It's quite frustrating to prepare food that you cannot eat — in fact many people find it difficult to even have their favorite foods in the house while on HCG — so think about what roles could shift for the time you're doing this important work. Ideally, anyone in the home who can reach the countertop would prepare their own meals, unless they're doing HCG with you.

We've heard frustrations from patients who say that they worked hard to prepare special dishes for themselves while on HCG and a roommate, partner or child ate their food. Be clear with others in your home that you have relatively few choices for the next few months. If they are choosing to eat what they normally eat, they should not also help themselves to the few things you can have right now. Failing this, there's the hide-it-in-aluminum-foil trick. Few housemates will bother to investigate something at the back of the fridge or freezer that is wrapped in foil and labeled "liver and onions."

Figuring out kitchen roles is important because in all, you'll probably be hyper-focused on what you can eat for about 2-3 months. You'll have two loading days + 21-40 very low calorie days + 2-3 weeks of Phase 3, slowly increasing your calories. It gets much easier in Phase 3, but you are still being very watchful and strategic.

During Phase 3, you'll have the opportunity to test for food sensitivities, which would extend the length of your diet, and some people extend P3 further still if they've had trouble stabilizing their weight in the past. It may help for everyone to know the timeline: there will be several months of housemates needing to keep their paws off your fish kebabs.

If someone close to you is tapping their foot while you work on your health, waiting impatiently for you to "get back to eating normally," you will notice it. If so, there may be larger themes in the relationship. For the time being, just focus on communicating what will be different in the kitchen for a few months.

People who live solo still have to communicate about what they will and won't do — there are work events, parties, coffee dates, happy hours, holidays, birthdays and fast food drive-through in our lives. People expect us to eat the way we did last the time they saw us.

Roles may shift for the positive, too. Don't forget to express your appreciation to anyone who is supportive of you. Let them know if you notice their adaptability, effort, good humor or warmth.

Ask for modest changes

Some patients tell us there's no way for them to avoid cooking non-HCG meals, due to the inability or unwillingness of others in the home to prepare their own meals. Asking for a few small, specific changes will increase your chances of success despite this.

— You might ask that foods you can't eat right now be put in the freezer, given to a food bank, brought to a potluck, given to friends or stored at a friend's house temporarily.

— You might ask that people not eat your favorite foods in your presence.

— You might ask that you still eat meals together, but that any adult who wants non-HCG food purchase those groceries him or herself.

— You might ask an adult who wants non-HCG food to order take-out meals. That take-out food should be consumed all at once if it's brought into the home; no tempting General Tso's Chicken leftovers in the refrigerator.

— You might ask that an adult who wants non-HCG food eat those meals out. He or she could still keep you company while you eat at home, if you both want that. Many people who have another adult in the house find this to be a simple solution. It's not done angrily, it's just pragmatic.

— You might cook a big enough HCG dish that you can render two versions: one that's simple, for you, and one that's more decadent, for someone else. For example, if you made an HCG **chicken and celery stir fry with Thai chiles**, you could separate some for yourself. Then **turn the rest into cashew chicken** for other people by adding sesame oil and toasted cashews and serving over rice.

— You could ask that the other(s) make their portion more decadent for themselves. *They* could be the ones to add sesame oil, cashews and rice to your HCG chicken stir fry to make it something they would enjoy.

Here's the thing: most people want to be thought of as "supportive" but not everyone knows what that looks like. Give them very specific examples of things they could do, like those above, that would be supportive.

Transitions reveal character

Some people find that their relationships are clarified when they do something good for themselves. Partners, children, siblings, friends, co-workers whom you hadn't imagined would pay much attention at all may rise to the occasion in beautiful ways. People can be incredibly thoughtful and funny and invested in ways we'd never seen before. Some of the people in your life may extend themselves in ways you'd not have imagined, ask how they can help you, share their admiration for your hard work or share their own experiences as a show of empathy. Transitions reveal good character.

Transitions reveal poor character, as well. In a few cases, people you felt close to, who have said, *"...You know I'll always be there for you..."* do not actually come through. Their motivations are more lazy or self-centered or just plain mean than you had realized. Transitions reveal pleasant surprises and unpleasant ones.

The examples of unpleasant surprises we hear from patients — about someone they thought would be supportive but wasn't — fall into several categories:

1. What you are asking of them presents an inconvenience they are not willing to undertake. They want everything to be as they have arranged it for themselves up to this point. Making changes, for you, is not appealing.

2. Your attention to new, healthy choices pulls focus away from them. They have become accustomed to you being aware of their needs and making that a priority. They had not imagined equal attention to your needs, even for a few months.

3. Your being proactive is a switch they do not appreciate. They think of themselves as the one who is powerful, the one who makes important decisions, has dreams, follows through with plans. Your taking action feels like a challenge to their status.

4. Your diet gets them thinking about their own health, which is uncomfortable. They may assume that you are judging their weight, smoking, drinking. If not that, perhaps they privately feel anxious about changes they should be making. Either way, the result may be irritability towards your diet or withdrawal from any discussion of it.

To discover that someone is *not* "...always there for you..." when the chips are down is a startling realization. It can be quite upsetting to finally see the relationship so clearly. Some people find that when they are preparing for and undertaking HCG is a nice time to be in therapy.

Seeing your relationships more clearly is not the only reason therapy is well-timed to HCG. Deciding to lose weight is thought-provoking. There's emotional risk that your body might change and emotional risk that it might not. Our present life is related to our past experiences and to the trajectory we're on for the future. As obvious as this may seem, there are people who think that the most effective way to deal with the present is to "stay in the present." Nope. That's not how our minds work.

Cognitive Self-Assessment

Our mind can lead us to inaccurate assumptions at times. In fact, there are quite specific ways we tend to misperceive things. The way we each misinterpret information is part of our personal, cognitive style.

Inaccurate assumptions or **cognitive distortions** fuel anxiety and depression. These assumptions are unconscious. Even people who are highly rational have a few distortions to the way they interpret the world; that's just how it is. Cognitive distortions aren't crazy, but they can make life more difficult than necessary at times.

For this reason, it's useful to look at what *our particular* cognitive distortions are when trying to make some sort of change. *Making unconscious patterns into conscious thoughts is an opportunity to take action; to catch patterns and interrupt them.* Obviously, gaining these insights would be useful to you well beyond HCG!

Many of the categories on the list of cognitive distortions will not describe you at all. Each of us has a *few* cognitive distortions that are our typical style, our go-to interpretation of life when we're dealing with an ambiguous situation.

SELF-ASSESSMENT OF COGNITIVE DISTORTIONS

Which of the categories below describe the assumptions you're likely to make when you're on edge or don't have complete information? Your selections aren't about how you *always* think, they're about where your mind goes when you're uncomfortable.

Most people find that several of these cognitive distortions describe their style pretty well when they are uncertain about someone or something. If none of these describe you, is there some other way you tend to jump to conclusions?

All-or-Nothing Thinking
You tend to see things in black-or-white categories. If someone falls short of perfection, they failed. People are winners or losers, attractive or unattractive, strong or weak, with you or against you. This raises the emotional stakes quite high when anyone is imperfect.

Over-Generalization
You perceive a single, unpleasant event as evidence of an overall pattern. Not getting selected for a particular job feels like "...No one will ever hire me..." What you've experienced is a disappointment, not a pattern, but your mind over-generalizes, so it already feels like a pattern.

Mental Filter
You notice a single, negative detail and dwell upon it. Your entire sense of reality becomes tainted by this one negative observation. Only noticing negative details blocks positive information from making an impression, so your reality becomes imbalanced.

Denying the Positive
You dismiss positive experiences when they occur, insisting they don't count. You idealize someone else's strengths but overlook your own. You can't take credit for your accomplishments. You always find some reason that something good about you isn't

really that good. By denying the positive, you maintain a negative self image not based in reality.

Catastrophizing

You accurately observe that something was unfair or someone was critical of you. (After all, sometimes when we assume someone doesn't like us, we are right!) The problem is the weight you assign this observation. The event was unpleasant, but you consider it awful. The unpleasant event feels like a catastrophe that will take time to recover from.

Mind-Reading

Assuming you know what someone else is thinking or feeling and having an emotional reaction to that. This not only causes unnecessary anger, hurt and anxiety, it can prevent you from actually asking that person what they are thinking. You are responding to a *guess* about someone else's intentions.

Fantasy

You have imagined how future events will turn out in such vivid detail that it actually feels as though those things have happened. What you have imagined feels so real that you have trouble getting grounded; it's hard to remember that these things have not actually occurred and you don't need to defend against them.

Emotional Reasoning

Mistaking your emotional reactions for what defines reality. For instance, believing, "... *If I feel offended, she must have been offensive...*" or "*...If I feel hurt, he was being hurtful...*" or "*...If that rule feels biased to me, it was unfair...*" Emotional reasoning means that you have trouble considering other perspectives when you're hurt or angry. If it felt bad to you, you assume it was in fact bad.

Unreasonable Demands

Expecting yourself to feel the way you believe people *should feel* in this situation. For example, feeling guilty about doing something for yourself because you've been taught that it's selfish. Following these commands prevents you from figuring out what you actually think or feel. (Proud or relieved, perhaps?) Our unreasonable demands may be directed at other people, too. This leads to resentment when they don't agree that they *should* feel something specific (responsible, thoughtful or appreciative, for example).

Labeling

Attaching a label to someone who made a single mistake, as if it's a lifelong trait. If you lose your keys occasionally you label yourself "absent-minded." Someone arrives late due to car trouble and you now regard them "unreliable." Labeling is calling yourself or someone else a name when a less harsh interpretation would have worked fine.

Personalization

Taking things more personally than is necessary, without having gathered information. Being easily offended. For example, thinking you alone are being criticized when a whole group is getting feedback. Perceiving yourself as unlucky when what happened to you happens to a lot of people. Assuming someone declined an invitation because they don't respect you, when it may be for some other reason, and so on. Taking things personally is exhausting; not a good use of energy.

Insights about Cognitive Distortions

What's the point of taking an inventory of our cognitive distortions if we all have them? Because when we know how we think under stress, we can sometimes catch a pattern before it throws us off more than necessary. Most people trying to lose weight or maintain a loss have psyched themselves out many times. Having some insight about how our perception is distorted at times enables us to exercise more control.

Here's an example relevant to the HCG experience. Some people on the diet assume that they will be criticized or disliked for turning down food someone has else has made. They imagine that interaction in such detail, replaying it over and over in their mind, that they don't even try to be assertive about their dietary needs. They have given up in anticipation of something going wrong, even though it hasn't yet. That cognitive distortion is **Fantasy** because *imagining* a difficult situation in detail has undermined them in real life.

If that person now has awareness — that when nervous, they tend to imagine a scenario in such great detail that they treat it as though it were real — they may be able to head this off at the pass. Perhaps they will go to an event already feeling full and not eat anything. Or go and say no to food they can't eat. Perhaps they'll even tell friends in advance that they need to bring some of their own food.

If this person caught the cognitive distortion as it was happening, they could say to themselves "...It's certainly *possible* I will be criticized for turning down some foods. I don't know that in advance, but I can rehearse what I'll say if I'm faced with that situation. I will follow through with my plans no matter what, but will try not to hurt the other person...." In other words, they have an opportunity to change their self-talk and strategize; we all do.

Insight about our own cognitive distortions is also useful when anxiety or depression have become a bit much. It's common to dig ourselves in deeper than is necessary when thoughts become a runaway train. If you can analyze how your thoughts might be inaccurate you may be able to catch anxiety or depression and regain your sense of humor. It's amazing how nutty and self-critical our assumptions can be.

Of course, sometimes our fears are accurate. We imagine some comment is about us personally and it actually is. We worry that one thing going wrong is a sign that it's all headed that direction and it all does go that way. This exercise is not about assuming that all anxiety is a distortion; not at all. Anxiety is extremely important to our being cautious and productive. Examining cognitive distortions is just about trying to reduce the number of misperceptions we generate, so our emotional life is based in reality as much as possible.

Personal Insights Useful for Weight Loss

Most people understand that self-awareness increases the probability their behavior change will stick. Strangely, some people don't get this, though. They do want to avoid repeating old patterns but they don't understand how they perpetuate those patterns. Let's examine the connection between insight and positive outcomes when making a life change. Some people accomplish this with psychotherapy but there are also some questions you can ask yourself independently.

Go with your strengths

The weeks you are on HCG may be an odd time. Reflect upon the conditions that bring out the best in you and run with this knowledge as much as possible:

* How do you personally respond to challenging projects? By actively planning or by trying to relax and see how things will unfold?

* Do you prefer to keep a broad, organic vision of your success or to focus on detailed step-by-step goals that may produce the outcome you wish for?

* Do you feel motivated by setbacks or simply discouraged by them? Are you motivated by success or does it make you complacent?

* How willing are you to seek information when there's something you don't know? Do you prefer to skip past the parts that are unclear or do you explore the unknown?

The most important question to ask yourself regarding using your strengths on HCG:
Are you a person who does better with predictability, routine and clear instructions or with variety, novelty and decision-making? This will determine how you approach meals during your time on Phase 2.

For those who love predictability

If you prefer the structure of food lists and the clarity of precise recipes, do your meal planning accordingly. Many people feel more secure by developing a routine than they do making multiple decisions. If you wish, don't worry about seeking new ingredients and calculating their carbs or protein, just go with our lists of suggested fruit, vegetables and proteins. You might chart what you'll have at each meal and what ingredients you will need to accomplish this. Perhaps breakfast is the same every weekday. Perhaps dinner is fish on Monday, Wednesday and Friday. Keep pre-portioned meals in the fridge and freezer. Go with your strengths.

You do best with routine and clear instruction

If you are the kind of person who is most likely to succeed on P2 by knowing what you will have to eat at each meal, with no calculations to make on-the-fly and no coming up blank for ideas, organization will be your greatest strength.

Interestingly, many people say that planning their menu in advance is quite helpful when on HCG, even if they typically like a lot of variety in their diet. Perhaps it reduces suffering to limit the decision-making, just like having a personal trainer pre-determine how many push-ups you'll do that day. Even if organization is not your super power, you may find it less torturous to plan than to improvise.

For example, if you don't love fish but you have determined that every Wednesday night you'll eat halibut (because you can eat lots of it) then just get on with it. You can make roast **blackened Cajun halibut,** or make it the star of a **saffron bouillabaisse,** or bake it in a **parchment packet with bok choy,** but on Wednesdays you'll have halibut for dinner. If you prefer, make it the exact same dish every Wednesday with the exact same portion size.

Go through this book and identify dishes that appeal to you, then assure you have those ingredients on hand. Do the self-assessment in the section on Cognitive Distortions, then do some thinking or writing about the assumptions that undermine you personally. Review the Twenty Preparations chapter.

Create a logistics grid: "...This week, my lunch every day will be a **shrimp salad on butter lettuce and radicchio with an MCT lime vinaigrette.** I take it with me to work in a big plastic bowl with a tight lid that I wash every night. I will make a week's worth of vinaigrette and use 2 tablespoons each day...."

Enter your entire *shrimp salad with lime vinaigrette* meal on the MyFitnessPal app under "My Meals," so you'll never need to enter those ingredients separately again. For every meal you determine that you're happy with, enter it as a meal rather than as individual ingredients; this will make your tracking very efficient.

Other organization tips: Defrost your freezer and make room for new P2 dishes you prepare. Cook in bulk. Put dishes in well-labeled, individual containers. Grow herbs on your windowsill. Make flavored iced teas the day before you need them. Hard boil some eggs and have the whites ready to go in a bowl with a spice mix you can shake on them.

If you are in the "I want clear instructions" camp, consider making a move towards choosing your own foods based upon protein density and carbohydrate count. This isn't just an exercise in improvisation, it's more effective for fat loss than following the original protocol to the letter is.

What you may need to *work on* if routine is your style

— Understanding the science behind food choices, so you will not become superstitious about why the diet works.

— Trying to use the calculations we describe to add a few ingredients to your repertoire.

— Not damaging your metabolism by eating fewer calories than recommended.

— Not assuming if you plateau that it's because you did something wrong.

For those who love variety

Personal decision-making about what to eat makes the diet much easier for some people; it makes them less likely to feel deprived or to rebel. That's why the original 1954 HCG protocol works much better for some people than others.

You are happier with degrees of freedom and don't mind the work of making decisions. You feel confident that you can make intelligent choices. You are inspired by the opportunity to create flavor while losing weight efficiently. You know that staying away from rigid food lists will increase your success. To go with that strength, get yourself out to ethnic markets. Incorporate the cooking ideas presented here. Provide yourself as many HCG-safe options as possible.

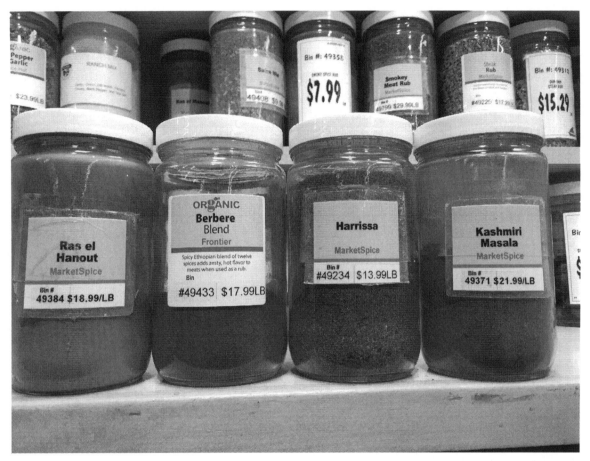

Photo: Dana Falk

North African and Middle Eastern spices offer tremendous, complex flavor; just a sprinkle can elevate something that's plain, like egg whites or cauliflower. Many of these are spice blends, not single origin spices, so check the label for any sugar that appears high on the list of ingredients.

You do best with novelty and independent choices

If you are the kind of person who is most likely to succeed on P2 with food that tastes really good and meals that are not repetitive, your strength will be creativity and adaptability. You'll go shopping for interesting ingredients. You will have herbs and spices you've found at ethnic markets. You'll select meat and seafood based upon the protein density score and your interest in them, not based on the original HCG protocol. You'll select veggies based upon their carb count and flavor as well as by how versatile they are in your kitchen. If you don't like the taste of something you made, you will toss it and invent something new. If it's midnight and you need **fresh spinach for an egg white omelette** in the morning, you'll go get spinach.

Pushing a little past our favored style serves us well in life. *If you are in the "Don't give me too many rules" camp, remember that doing it the way other people do it doesn't steal your soul.* You can still be creative in your cooking while observing guidelines. You can follow a protocol without losing your individuality.

What you may need to *work on* if variety is your style

— Following instructions for calories, carbs, water, etc. Don't rely upon memory.

— Making sure you have arranged grab-and-go foods for car, bag and work, even if they're ordinary.

— Having too many treats or too much sweetener.

— Spending too much time in the kitchen, still obsessing over food.

A taste of honey

Here's another example of knowing your strengths, as a practical matter. Do you sustain changes more effectively when you allow yourself a little bit of the things you love or when you entirely rule out certain foods?

Some people go off the rails once they start eating something they love and they have difficulty stopping. For these people, getting a taste of honey (literally or figuratively) is a bad idea. Other people go off the rails when they feel deprived of the foods they love. For these people, it's better to have a nibble of something they love (even when on HCG) than it is to rule a favorite food out entirely. Take stock of whether you should allow yourself treats or not.

To use an HCG Phase 2 example: some people find that allowing themselves a little mango, which is very high in carb count but very delicious, keeps them from feeling deprived and over-reacting. If they can suck on a few cubes of frozen mango or leave a slice floating in their water jug or mash a little mango as a topping for mahi mahi, they can stay on the program. Other people have a tendency to binge once they get a taste of something yummy. Mango, with its sweet/acidic flavor profile, is very high in fructose (as are most tropical fruits). That could trigger physiological cravings that spark a week of eating mango. The cravings might even broaden to include other fruits or all sweets.

In short, knowing your personality is quite useful. Plan for a few treats if *that* plays to your strengths. Clean your house of all temptations if *that* plays to your strengths.

The context of childhood

No matter how old we are now, the beliefs instilled in us when we were young are perfectly relevant to how we think, feel and act today. Even if we disagree with the messages our family was sending us about the value of self-improvement — heck, even if we *knew as a child* that we disagreed with their position — we're wired to care about what our family thinks. Now that you're trying to do something good for your health, it's possible you'll have some of those family attitudes on your mind. So let's take a look at the context of your childhood home.

How was self-improvement regarded in your original family?

— Was it active, as in *"That sounds great. What can we do to help?"*
— Was it supportive, as in *"Good for you!"*
— Was it spirited, as in *"Great idea. Let's all do that together!"*
— Was it optimistic, as in *"...You can accomplish anything you undertake."*
— Was it passive, as in *"If it's meant to be, it will happen."*
— Was it disengaged, as in *"Sure, if you want to do that, go ahead."*
— Was it competitive, as in *"Let's see if you can do that as well as _____ does."*
— Was it defeatist, as in *"Why bother? We are who we are."*
— Was it shaming, as in *"You should have done that a long time ago."*
— Was demeaning, as in *"You think you're so important that we should all adjust?"*
— Was it hurtful, as in *"You've tried that before and failed."*

Here are some ways our childhood family attitudes towards self-improvement are still relevant to how we think in adulthood:

— Some people had warm, supportive families who were always rooting for them. They now feel embarrassed that they have not been able to make changes, despite this encouragement.

— Some people noticed their family's ineffectiveness with self-improvement. As adults, there's now a deep hopelessness that prevents them from pursuing happiness or change.

— Some people were expected to improve upon everything they did when they were a kid. The family was gung-ho, high energy. As an adult, they have been avoiding self-improvement for years. They may be more calm or more introverted than the rest of their family is.

— Some people had very encouraging, loving family attitudes towards self-improvement but they weren't taught any skills for success. They desire self-improvement but don't know how to work towards it, because the family was a bit disorganized or didn't understand that there are skills involved in goal-setting.

— Some people had very kind families that were passive or depressive. The kids weren't discouraged from self-care, but the parent(s) weren't lifting the kids up or lifting themselves up. Everyone was getting by fine, but not making progress. Now, as an adult, you have to figure it out on your own if you want change.

— Some people came from achievement-oriented families. Everyone was driven towards self-improvement and seemed great at making things happen. The family's confidence felt a bit overwhelming then and feels a bit overwhelming now.

— Some people had a family in distress. They have no idea what the attitudes towards self-improvement were, because there was no room for that sort of thing. Worry about personal goals is not on the table if conflict, financial need, physical and sexual safety, abandonment or chaos is a concerns.

What we learn about our family's attitudes towards self-improvement isn't usually stated directly; we have to decode it. For example, if the family climate was, *"You make us proud no matter what you do,"* that was probably conveyed with warmth rather than words. If the family climate was, *"Who you are as an individual isn't important. Just make us look good,"* it's unlikely those words were spoken directly. Values are subtle; they're communicated by way of what behaviors are rewarded with attention and affection and what behaviors are punished with disdain, criticism or no response at all.

If you see your family described here, or you don't, but seeing these examples helps you clarify what the family culture was, you now have a tool to work with. You may now define your own, adult attitudes towards self-care. If you have admiration for what you learned about self improvement as a child, you may wish to work harder towards these ideals. If you disagree with what you learned, you may prepare to undertake life goals differently.

To be clear, it's not that we're made perfect by a healthy family dynamic or irreversibly screwed-up by an unhealthy one. It's just that being tuned-in to the context we grew up with helps us understand the hopes, skills and expectations we bring to any big project. Losing weight is a big, important, emotional project.

As you move into this important project, ask yourself more about the context of your childhood:

— Is there something very positive someone in your family does when taking on challenges that you would like to emulate?

— Is there something your family believed about body image you need to disregard?

— Is there anything you learned about the importance of self esteem or hard work that was inspiring?

— Is there anything you over-react to because you're remembering criticism?

— Have you developed a pattern of giving up on past self-improvement projects that your family now assumes you will repeat? Can you set this aside and focus on the task at hand?

— Is there a special skill you learned in your family that you could make use of right now?

Combat all-or-nothing thinking

All-or-nothing thinking is one of the most important distortions to keep an eye on, as anyone who has ever tried to lose weight will attest to. It's that tendency to think you had either a "good eating day" or a "bad eating day." It's the tendency to keep a score card and consider the day wasted if we're not happy with how we ate after dinner, even if our eating the rest of that day was brilliant.

If you recall, cognitive distortions are about how we freak out a little when we have incomplete information; how we fill in the gaps with assumptions that may not be accurate. Being on HCG is one of those times that we have incomplete information. If the scale stalls for a day or two, you don't quite know how that happened. Is it because you made a mistake the day before or because your body is taking a breather before it releases more weight?

How to combat all-or-nothing thinking while on HCG:
If you have eaten something you regret, pick yourself up and dust yourself off. Your body doesn't know what day of the week it is, so you haven't "blown the day." There's no sense in deciding "I've ruined this day. I'll re-start HCG tomorrow morning."

Try thinking of the day as divided into four quarters. If you're unhappy with what you ate mid-morning (Quarter 1), keep calm and carry on for a good showing in the afternoon (Quarter 2) and the early evening (Quarter 3). Some people eat well all day then overeat at night (Quarter 4). That means you'll concentrate harder tomorrow on Quarter 4; it doesn't wipe away your successful eating Quarters 1-3. This cognitive approach to pushing past all-or-nothing-thinking works well for any kind of change you might be making, not just for eating habits.

Feeling completely defeated due to one fumble would be experiencing your mistake out of proportion to its actual cost. HCG is not an all-or-nothing enterprise; neither is healthy eating beyond HCG and neither is life in general.

Success and failure both cause anxiety

People who have never been overweight might assume that being slender would feel completely amazing and that failing to lose weight would feel crushing. In reality, it's far more complex than that. People who have always been slender may not understand the psychological benefits of being larger and the anxieties that are natural to becoming slender.

It's very common to fear success as much as we fear failure. People aren't always aware of their fear of success though: it requires special insight.

Broker a deal for treats

Because our bodies over-react to eating the wrong thing when on the HCG hormone, the stakes are higher than normal. This is fact, not fiction. The intensity makes some people feel invigorated, some feel deprived. When we feel deprived we're at higher risk of backsliding.

You can use this insight to decide that you'll make something a little special for yourself, but something that's not self-destructive. Broker a deal with yourself for a treat that will prevent bigger problems. Perhaps this would mean having a larger portion of a P2 protein (extra meatballs) or eating a protein with a poorer protein density (dark meat chicken instead of white meat). It might mean making a P2 dish with something extra tasty added (a little apple in your slow cooker pork or a few beans in your chili). To prevent backsliding, it's best you not feel overly deprived.

Let's try an example of brokering a deal with yourself. We know that drinking a typical milkshake made with ice cream and chocolate sauce would have real consequences for you while on HCG. What if, instead, you made yourself an **extra thick, extra chocolatey whey protein shake?** Give yourself a big, heaping scoop of protein powder to make the shake thicker, a tablespoon of good, unsweetened cocoa powder (even if the whey protein is chocolate flavor) to make it taste richer. Then add some vanilla extract and a pinch of salt to make the flavor more complex.

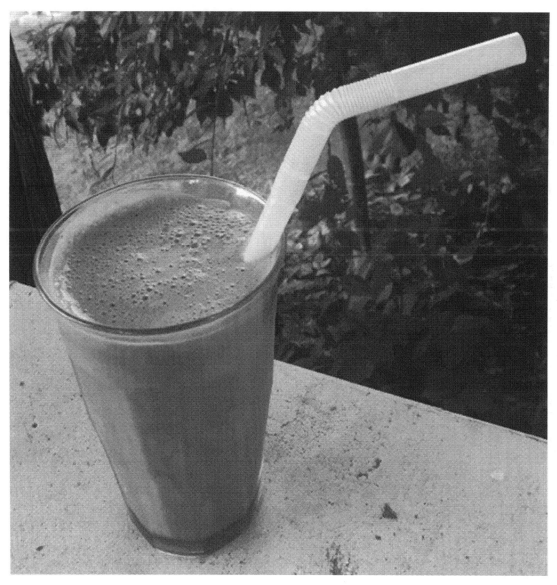

Photo: Dana Falk

You'll get good at making treats that satisfy a craving but don't do damage to your progress. Go for extra taste or a larger portion rather than adding sugar, starch or fat. This chocolate whey protein shake has 1 tbs unsweetened cocoa powder + 1 pinch salt for depth of flavor. This shake was made with 16 ice cubes and 1/2 cup coffee. For the consistency of soft serve ice cream, decrease the liquid you add and increase the ice cubes.

Whip up this HCG-safe milkshake instead of a real milkshake and you have problem-solved very well! You've invested a few more calories but made an HCG food extra satisfying. Sure, it might mean you go over your target calories for the day, but *this is strategic, it's not backsliding.* You avoided all-or-nothing thinking by brokering a deal with yourself.

No Shame in Quitting

Some of us were taught that we should always finish what we start, that hardship builds character, that bailing on something is shameful even if it was never a good fit to begin with. Some families, teachers, friends and communities teach us that quitting makes you a "quitter." Mental health professionals often disagree with this philosophy.

Sticking around no matter what results in people remaining in unhealthy jobs, relationships, hobbies and environments to the point of misery, or at least to the point of being counter-productive. People who refuse to quit are not always heroes. *People who stop doing something that's counter-productive are not "quitters."*

Where the HCG Diet is concerned, if you realize that the very low calorie phase isn't healthy for you — that the deprivation makes you binge, for example, or that you over-do caloric restriction and slip into not eating at all — ending your round may be the most intelligent choice. It's counter-productive to work hard at something that's pulling you farther away from your ultimate goal.

Here's the insight exercise to try: Are you really following the plan? How honest are you with your healthcare provider about what you're up to? Keeping notes, a spreadsheet or a journal is a good way of tracking your responses to the HCG *process*, not just the outcomes. You may actually know the answers to these questions without hard data.

Don't be critical of yourself if you decide to step away from the HCG Diet. From our perspective, a quitter is someone who has a long-standing pattern of dropping things they can't master quickly. Evaluating whether something is helping or hurting you, on a case-by-case basis, is an entirely different matter. That is called realistic self-appraisal, and in mental health terms, it's the ideal.

Why People Fear Weight Loss

To increase your chances of accomplishing your goals on HCG, give some thought to whether you might have some reservations about significant weight loss for any of these reasons:

— Some people would be embarrassed to lose weight because they believe it would be admitting that they were unhappy before.

— Some people look upon losing weight as giving in to societal expectations or gender role conventions.

— Some people have a partner who is overweight and worry they'd be abandoning that person if they were no longer overweight along with them.

— Some people imagine they will never be able to eat tasty food again if they lose weight. They decide that they would rather "enjoy life" and not lose weight.

— Some people have an identity that's about helping other people maximize *their* potential. It feels odd to be pursuing their own goals.

— Some people despise exercise. They assume they would have to exercise if they wanted to keep weight off (FYI, exercise is helpful but not required for maintaining weight loss.)

— Some larger people don't have much respect for slender people. They see them as less brave, less interesting, less sensual.

— Some people have lost weight and gained it back before; they worry that they will just confirm their usual pattern to themselves and others.

— Some people worry that friends and family would be a little too enthusiastic about their weight loss. It would feel as though other people had been waiting a long time for this to happen, but had been holding their tongue.

— Some people have had a person telling them they *should* lose weight. Actually doing so feels like giving in.

— Some people have their identity tied to being larger, such as being a powerful person, an athlete, a funny person, a self-sacrificing person or an independent thinker.

— Some people believe that a thin cook is not a good cook, or that any sophisticated "foodie" would not be slender.

— Some people associate being slender with unwanted sexual attention.

— Some people believe it would be impractical to lose weight, since they would have to buy an entirely new wardrobe and such.

— Some people worry that a partner will emotionally abuse them for being "selfish."

— Some people sense that weight loss will require too much effort; if they give up early, they can relax.

— Some people want to decrease the chances of being expected to date or to socialize. They are actually just introverted, but use their size as an opportunity to isolate.

— Some people worry that once they feel better about themselves, they will really notice when they are not being treated well.

— Some people miss a loved one who was overweight and has passed away. They believe that becoming slender would make them feel more distant from that loved one. (Usually this fear is unconscious.)

— Some people are concerned that working to lose weight will take time away from more important things.

— For some people, being large is quite common within their cultural or regional community. They worry that changing their own body might be viewed as rejecting their community or thinking they are superior.

— Some people have always been overweight and wonder if that's simply what's meant to be for their lifetime.

— For some people, being plus size has gotten them out of doing things they never wanted to do in the first place; their size serves a purpose.

— Some people are aware that being overweight may shorten their life, but privately that's what they wish for. (The same is true for heavy drinking, smoking, etc.)

— Some people think success [of any kind] is showy or egotistical.

— Some people fear that success with their weight in adulthood will make them more aware of missed opportunities across their life: a career they didn't pursue, not having children when they could, not buying a place when the neighborhood was affordable.

— For some people, body image and weight loss efforts have been a constant worry for years; practically their hobby. Getting it done might feel like a loss.

— Some people are happier with struggle. Success feels dull, like an ending.

If any of these concerns strike a chord for you, it may help explain why your past efforts to lose weight have been ineffective or temporary. Perhaps there was something genuinely scary about losing weight. If you want this time around to be different, you now know where to focus your energy.

FYI, fear of success is a human issue that goes well beyond body image. Many people in therapy discuss their anxiety about career promotions, happy relationships, financial success and other things you might assume they are comfortable with. We don't just worry about losing, we worry about winning.

Food as a Lifelong Issue

Of all the sensual things people use for comfort or escape, food may be the toughest to manage. Unlike tobacco, alcohol, sex, exercise, caffeine, opioids, video games, pot, gambling, porn, cleaning, hoarding or any other way we soothe ourselves, giving up eating is not an option. We cannot live without food, so we must reckon with it.

If you have achieved better perspective on your relationship with food through HCG, that's a serious win. If you have improved on health biomarkers other than weight, like blood sugars, liver health, inflammation, insulin resistance, food sensitivities, acid reflux, blood pressure, complexion or leptin sensitivity, that's *incredibly* impressive. Bear in mind how many benefits there are to metabolic health, because food may be a lifelong issue.

In her book *Weight-Loss Apocalypse* (2011), Robin Phipps Woodall notes the importance of compulsive eaters developing a genuine desire to eat less, independent of weight loss as a reward for that. That's hard to imagine for someone who has been a compulsive eater most of his or her life! Woodall believes that finding natural moderation with food requires people to be accountable for their emotions. If people find happiness beyond food, she says, moderation comes naturally. She's probably right. Many patients find that reading *Weight-Loss Apocalypse* is helpful for understanding how they became a compulsive eater and the work it may take to prevent it from becoming a lifelong theme.

How to overcome compulsive eating

Not everyone who loves food is compulsive about it, but for many people, moderation will always be a challenge. It's not just a love of *eating*, right? It's a passion for so many other aspects of food: trying new restaurants, watching cooking shows, creating your own recipes, entertaining friends, learning about culture from cuisine, seeking hard-to-find ingredients and appreciating the very best version of any dish. If that's you, whether you consider yourself a "foodie" or not, managing love of food may be a lifelong project. You may always be working to strike a balance between living a good, tasty life and thinking too much about food, even once you're happy with your physical health.

In essence, compulsive eating is about using factors other than hunger to determine when and how much we eat. One way to overcome this is to master noticing how hungry you are when you begin to eat and how full you are when you stop eating. Details below!

During HCG Phases 2 and 3 is not the right time to hone these skills, because you may not have the luxury of eating whenever you're hungry or enjoying portions that make you full. As you *complete* Phase 3 and are looking to life beyond, that's the perfect time to work on understanding hunger cues.

Hunger Rating Scale

To address compulsive eating, practice rating your hunger on this scale of 1-10

1   =   So hungry you feel desperate; constant hunger.

2   =   Feeling very hungry. Strong hunger pangs.

3   =   Noticing you're quite hungry, actively seeking food.

4   =   Getting hungry, ready for a bite.

5   =   Not hungry, but not full. Hard to tell if satisfied.

6   =   Getting satisfied, but still have appetite. Prefer to eat more.

7   =   Pleasantly satisfied.

8   =   Feeling full.

9   =   So full it's unpleasant; feeling stuffed, bloated, tired.

10   =   So full you feel sick or in pain.

It takes practice to tune-in to hunger with such specificity; most of us are not paying such close attention. Here, you're being asked to (1) pay attention to hunger cues and (2) use a system that anchors intensity of hunger to reliable points on a scale. It's taking something that's usually abstract, like our appetite, and making it quantifiable. That is a skill and it's not easy.

Step-by-step use of hunger ratings

1. Your first task is to get very familiar with the hunger rating scale. Understand the meaning of each point on the scale and re-write the description of any point you don't like. To understand the ends of the spectrum, think about whether you have ever felt Level 1 or Level 10. Work on memorizing the scale well enough that you could rate your hunger level without referring to the list.

2. Next, practice noticing what Level 5 feels like; this is the most difficult point on the scale to master. Take some notes each time you believe you are at Level 5 hunger. What were the signs that pointed to feeling neutral? Some patients say they know they're at a 5 when they can still get work done without planning a meal. Some say they know it because if they drink a few sips of a beverage, they feel satisfied. Figure out what your "tells" are.

It's important to be able to sense a neutral "not hungry, not full" state, because it's a dividing line. Compulsive eaters usually eat at a '5' and non-compulsive eaters usually do not. Non-compulsive eaters wait until they sense physical hunger, unless there's some special occasion. Compulsive eaters, on the other hand, take the absence of fullness to mean hunger.

If you really can't pinpoint what Level 5 hunger feels like, write detailed definitions for Level 4 and Level 6. You'll define Level 5 as any sensation that falls between these.

3. Make a note of where you are on the scale each time you start and stop eating. You're not trying to change these eating habits yet, just trying to track your current patterns. Can you use increments of 1/2, as in "My hunger is a 4.5 right now?" Sure. This all yields terrific information, so do it your way. Consider creating a spreadsheet or just having an easy way to jot this information on your phone or in a little notebook. Remember, you're not changing your eating in this step, just noting where you are each time you start and stop eating. Track for at least five days.

4. The next goal is to assure that you are at least a little hungry each time you begin to eat (4 or less on the hunger scale). Work on trying to change this habit until you're able to do it about 75% of the time. This may take days or it may take weeks.

Many of us have gotten into the habit of eating because food is available, rather than because we are hungry. Now you're being asked to wait until you feel something quite specific, so be patient with the process. This is a major attitude adjustment.

One trick some people use to get over the hump of waiting for hunger to eat is to tell themselves, "…If you wait until you're physically hungry, at Level 4 or lower, you may eat whatever you want, within reason…."

5. The next goal is to assure that you always stop eating before you become uncomfortably full (Level 8 or lower on the hunger scale.) Again, jot some notes. How do you know when you're moving from (7) *pleasantly full* to (8) *quite full?*

Some people say they know they are moving from 7 to 8 when the speed of their eating decreases. They end up at Level 8 if they keep taking bites of something because it tastes good, because it was expensive, because it's a special opportunity, etc., even though their appetite dropped off sharply at Level 7. Ideally, you'd stop eating at Level 7 on an average day and Level 8 when there's something super special or super tasty.

Once you've accomplished these tasks, you're no longer eating compulsively! Technically, if you are eating only when hungry and stopping once full, that's non-compulsive eating. You've really accomplished something at this point.

From here, you fine tune:

6. *In terms of appetite*, the ideal is to be hungry but not over-hungry when you begin to eat (Levels 2-3-4.) Some people stay away from Level 2 hunger, because it makes them want to binge. Some people dislike Level 4 hunger, because they want to challenge themselves to feel more than a little peckish before they eat. All this is a matter of knowing yourself. Being at Level 3 is probably the gold standard for non-compulsive eating, but waiting for hunger to go from Level 5 to 4 is challenge enough for most people who have overeaten in the past.

7. *In terms of fullness,* the ideal is to eat until you are satisfied or full but not stuffed (Levels 6-7-8.) Again, some people stay away form Level 6, because they do not want to feel hungry again too soon. Some people stay away from Level 8, because their goal is to never feel that full. This fine tuning is up to you. Perhaps stopping at Level 7 is the gold standard, but being able to reliably stop at a 6, 7 or 8 is fantastic for someone who has been an overeater.

8. An advanced experiment in non-compulsive eating: how much food does it take you to get from one level of hunger to the next? If you are a little hungry (Level 4) how much food does it take to just make the hunger go away? (Level 5). If you are super hungry (Level 2) how much do you have to eat to get to a more comfortable level of hunger? (Level 3). Often, it takes less food than we think it will to make hunger subside.

One patient told us that she conducted this experiment when she was at Level 2 hunger one morning. She was feeling quite ravenous for a large breakfast, but decided to play with the moment instead and see how little food it would require to take the edge off her hunger. She was shooting for Level 3 or 4 hunger. She ate a tablespoon of gruyere cheese and one-quarter of a small red bell pepper. This snack brought her from Level 2 to Level 4 hunger and that lasted for 1 hour, 15 minutes. During that time, she was focused on work and not feeling hungry. After 1 hour 15 minutes, she dropped down to Level 3, so became aware that she was hungry and began to seek food. She decided not to wait until she returned to Level 2 hunger, which was uncomfortable, and ate a normal-sized breakfast at Level 3. What a worthwhile experiment! She learned she didn't need to put much in her belly to make the growling stop. She also learned that she eats more reasonable meals when not overly hungry.

9. Another advanced experiment: Use your grounding in the hunger rating scale to prevent binges. When people get too hungry, they may eat aggressively to the point of being stuffed. Hunger that gets too intense can trigger feelings of deprivation and make us over-respond. If you ever get overly hungry and are tempted to binge, go back to your original notes to remind you what Level 8 feels like. That will be your goal, to eat to Level 8, but not 9 or 10. Eat until you're quite full, but not stuffed.

Beyond attuning to your level of hunger, another technique for avoiding over-eating is to always have a healthy snack with you, in case of emergency. Keep a meat stick, string cheese, **HighKey Snacks keto cheese crunch**, a cucumber, a **Keto Krisp bar,** a little packet of unsweetened almond butter, **Dang lightly salted coconut chips** or a **Dang Keto Bar,** some celery, jalapeño Spanish peanuts, **Heka Good cookies**, pumpkin seeds (or whatever you choose) on hand at all times. You know this trick already, but it takes some commitment to plan for actually having shelf stable, healthy snacks within reach at all times. Perhaps have a recurring order set up or buy in bulk when you find something you like.

It's unrealistic to expect ourselves to eat non-compulsively all day / every day. Even people with no real food issues sometimes eat for reasons other than hunger. Still, knowing how to work with your hunger is a powerful tool for life beyond HCG.

We wish you a happy, healthy relationship with food! Hoping you will continue to use the same creativity, strategy and insight you did with the HCG Diet throughout your life.

Use your foodie powers for good. We're rooting for you.

ACKNOWLEDGMENTS

With respect and affection for my mentors
Dr. Clara Hill, Dr. Arnie Medvene and Dr. Margaretha Lucas.
Their insight, intellect and generosity fostered my development
well beyond my years at Maryland.

— Dana Falk

With gratitude to my colleagues
Dr. Kim Celmer, Dr. Janci Karp and Dr. Genevieve Courtney,
who make me a better doctor every day
and to my patients, who bring such meaning and fulfillment to this work.

— Kelsey Klausmeyer

ABOUT THE AUTHORS

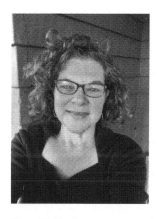 **Dana R. Falk, Ph.D.** is a Licensed Psychologist whose clinical specialties include adult transitions and anxiety. Dr. Falk has taught university courses in Processes of Change and graduate courses in Psychotherapy Skills.

Dr. Falk's research includes studies of laughter in psychotherapy, group therapy for divorce resilience and cross-cultural comparison of psychodynamic therapy in Argentina and the U.S.

Dr. Falk has received two Fulbright grants in Public Health: one to lecture on grief in Taiwan, the other PTSD outreach in Indonesia. Dr. Falk has also done freelance reporting on social issues for public radio stations WBEZ Chicago and KUOW Seattle.

Dr. Falk earned a Ph.D. in Counseling Psychology from the University of Maryland in 1993. She has been Chief Psychologist at a college health clinic and directed pre-doctoral internship training. Now in private practice, she continues to enjoy mentoring mental health professionals with clinical supervision.

Dr. Falk's approach to treatment integrates interpersonal, psychodynamic and cognitive behavioral therapies. She sees clients in Seattle, along with French Bulldog, Babette.

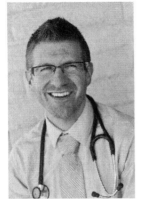 **Kelsey D. Klausmeyer, N.D.** is a Naturopathic Physician. Dr. Klausmeyer specializes in clinical management of weight loss for patients with weight loss resistance. He considers obesity a complex, chronic disease and evaluates infectious, metabolic, environmental, hormonal and genetic factors for underlying cause. He uses varied medical therapies such as diet plans, prescription medication and IV therapy.

Dr. Klausmeyer's scholarship includes body composition assessment, the pathophysiology of obesity and the science of novel interventions for obesity, such as the ketogenic diet. He has presented this work at national conferences.

Dr. Klausmeyer trains other naturopathic physicians and residents. He's been President of the Washington Association of Naturopathic Physicians and has served in the American Association of Naturopathic Physicians house of delegates. He's been a 'Top Doc' in Seattle Met magazine three times and his work was featured in the Seattle Times.

Dr. Klausmeyer earned a Doctorate of Naturopathic Medicine from Bastyr University in 2011. He practices at the Institute of Complementary Medicine in Seattle and is proud to serve the LGBTQ community.

REFERENCES

Brostoff, J. and Gamlin, L. (2000) *Food Allergies and Food Intolerance: The complete guide to their identification and treatment*. Healing Arts Press: Vermont.

Emmerich, M. and Emmerich, C. (2018) *Keto: The complete guide to success on the keto diet, including simplified science and no-cook meal plans*. Victory Belt Publishing: Las Vegas.

Freud, Sigmund (1951). *Psychopathology of Everyday Life*. New American Library: New York.

Fung, J. (2016) *The Obesity Code: Unlocking the Secrets of Weight Loss*. Vancouver/Berkeley: Greystone Books, pp 78-82.

Hallberg S.J., McKenzie, A.L., Williams P.T., Bhanpuri, N.H., Peters, A.L., Campbell, W.W., Hazbun, T.L., Volk, B.M., McCarter, J.P., Phinney, S.D. & Volek, J.S. (2018) *Effectiveness and Safety of a Novel Care Model for the Management of Type 2 Diabetes at One Year: An Open Label, Non-Randomized, Controlled Study*. Diabetes Therapy, 9(2): 583-612.

LaBoube, Z. (2013) *HCG 2.0: A Modern Adaptation of the Traditional HCG Diet*. Self-published: Amazon Digital Services.

Lam, R. (2015) *HCG Chica's HCG Diet Workbook*. Self-published: CreateSpace Independent Publishing Platform.

Martinez-Lopez, N., Tarabra, E., Toledo, M., Garcia-Macia, M., Sahu, S., Coletto, L., Batista-Gonzalez, A., Barzilai, N., Pessin, J., Schwartz, G., Sander, K. & Singh, R. (2017) *System Wide Benefits of Intermeal Fasting by Autophagy*. Cell Metabolism, 26 (6), 856-871.

McKenzie A.L., Hallberg, S.J., Creighton, B.C., Volk, B.M., Link, T.M., Abner, M.K., Glon, R.M., McCarter, J.P., Volek, J.S. & Phinney, S.D. (2017) *A Novel Intervention Including Individualized Nutritional Recommendations Reduces Hemoglobin A1c Level, Medication Use and Weight in Type 2 Diabetes.* JMIR Diabetes, 2(1):e5.

Northrup, C. (2012) The Wisdom of Menopause: Creating physical and mental health during the change. Bantam Books: New York.

Page, K. & Dornenburg, A. (2008) *The Flavor Bible: The essential guide to culinary creativity, based on the wisdom of America's most imaginative chefs.* Little, Brown and Company: New York.

Panda, S. (2018) *The Circadian Code.* Penguin Random House: New York. pp 94-121.

Patel, Y.R., Kirkman, M.S., Considine, R.V., Hannon, T.S. and Mather, K.J. (2016) *Changes in Weight and Glucose Can Protect Against Progression in Early Diabetes Independent of Improvements in-Cell Function.* J. of Clin Endocrinol Metab 101 (11) pp 4076-4084.

Phipps Woodall, R. (2011) *Weight-Loss Apocalypse: Emotional Eating Rehab Through the HCG Protocol.* Self-published: AuthorHouse.

Prochaska, J.O., Norcross, J.C. & DiClemente, C.C. (1994) *Changing for Good.* William Morrow and Company: New York, pp 174-176.

Rubin, G. (2015). *Better Than Before: Mastering the habits of our everyday lives.* Crown: New York.

Simeons, A.T.W. (1954) *Pounds and Inches: A new approach to obesity,* 7th ed., 2010. Popular Publishing: United States.

Steiner, J.L., Crowell, K.T. & Lang, C.H. (2015) *Impact of Alcohol on Glycemic Control and Insulin Action*, Biomolecules (5)4: 2223-2246.

Volek, J.S. & Phinney, S.D. (2012) *The Art and Science of Low Carbohydrate Performance.* Beyond Obesity, LLC: Createspace.com.

Made in the USA
Monee, IL
04 February 2021